Comfort
Heart

NATIONAL LIBRARY OF CANADA CATALOGUING IN PUBLICATION DATA

Cole, Carol Ann
Comfort heart: a personal memoir

ISBN 1-55022-473-5

1. Cole, Carol Ann. 2. Breast — Cancer — Patients — Biography. 3. Comfort Heart Initiative. 4. Women executives — Canada — Biography. I. Kapoor, Anjali II. Title.

RC280.B8C64 2001   362.1'9699449'0092   C2001-900811-2

Edited by Jennifer Hale
Cover and text design by Guylaine Régimbald – SOLO DESIGN
Front cover photo by Sue Mills
Back cover photo by Peter Sibbald
Author photo on page 179 by Matt Johannsson
Layout by Mary Bowness

Printed by Transcontinental

Distributed in Canada by
General Distribution Services,
325 Humber College Blvd.,
Toronto, ON M9W 7C3

Published by ECW PRESS
2120 Queen Street East, Suite 200
Toronto, ON M4E 1E2
ecwpress.com

This book is set in Electra and Runa.

PRINTED AND BOUND IN CANADA

The publication of *Comfort Heart* has been generously supported by the Canada Council, the Ontario Arts Council and the Government of Canada through the Book Publishing Industry Development Program. **Canadä**

Comfort Heart

A Personal Memoir

Carol Ann Cole

with
Anjali Kapoor

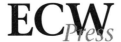

FOR JAMES

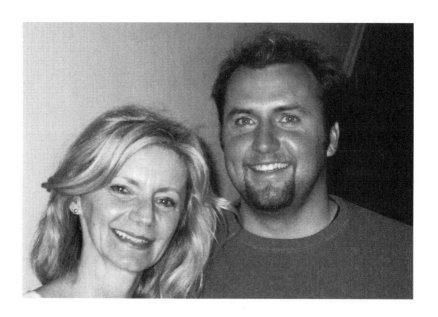

Table of Contents

Acknowledgements

So many people have said to me, "You really should write a book." I have talked about it for years. When I retired in 1994 and shared with Danny Bell that I was working on a book he asked me what it would be about. After replying, "I can't decide if it should be about my life or my career," Danny said without hesitation, "As I recall from when we were dating, your life and your career were one and the same." I have never forgotten his words and as I was writing this particular section of my book I contacted Danny to share with him that his comment had influenced my life, that I wanted to quote him in my book, and to thank him for being so honest with me. That's when he told me he had cancer; he had just been diagnosed. His courageous battle was a brief one, and sadly we lost Danny before I had the chance to thank him in print — thank you Danny.

When Al sent me this note after reading about the Comfort Heart Initiative in the *Bell News* he had no idea how successful the fund-raiser would become. He also did not know of my dream to write a book:

> Carol Ann
>
> Your friends at Bell are so proud of you + we all miss you. When it comes to heart you wrote the book.
>
> all the best
>
> al sty

I have so many people to thank.

First, to the man who is my friend, my confidant, and my son — James. Without your support and love for more than thirty years, I would not be the person I am today. I love you and I thank you for showing me that dreams do come true and for allowing me to grow up with you. To Tracey who completes your life, a very special thank you.

I owe so much to my sisters Lois, Lorraine, and Connie who undersood my need to write this book and continue to support me in all that I do. I am so fortunate to have sisters who are also my friends and I love you so much. Thank you to Tom and John for the exceptional way you carry out your "brother-in-law" duties!

To my relatives one and all — while it is true that we don't choose our relatives, I can honestly say I am proud to be related to each and every one of you. We collectively bring different things to the family and I think our many differences have helped me through my own journey. I hope you will recognize a tiny bit of yourself in my story and I thank you for the role you have played in my life.

Thank you to the thousands of "Holders of the Heart." I have said many times the Comfort Heart Initiative is not about me, but about all those who have helped me make a difference. I wish I could re-gift every award and recognition I have received to my many supporters. I am as grateful to individuals like Jack Fitzgerald, Trish Ress, Maureen Proctor, Nancy Archibald, Cheryl Munroe, and Cathy Connelly who continue to sell Comfort Hearts one at a time as I am for the corporate support my fund-raiser continues to enjoy. Thank you to Ruth Foster and the Bell Canada team, John Mach and my friends at Comtech Credit Union, Judy Charette, JC Legault and the Nexacor team, Hazel Gillespie and the Petro-Canada team, and so many others. Thank you to David Harland and Francis MacNamara who were the first to have Comfort Hearts available in their retail store, Yes.Ter.Year Interior Accents — I have used your example with many other businesses who are trying to decide if they want to "get involved."

May Ocean, Linda Power, and the OceanArt team continue to give me their total support and have shared my excitement about the completion of this book. I first met May and Linda when the Comfort Heart Initiative began and it now seems we have been life-long friends. You truly do share my dream! Thank you for selling so many Comfort Hearts, for carrying them with you to your many events so they can easily be available to the public, and thanks in advance for the many copies of my book I know you will sell!

I will forever be thankful to my lifelong friends Donna Cummings and Phyllis Pedicelli who continue to play a part in my life, and allow me to share theirs. Additionally, Al Peppard and my friends in Middleton as well as my Acadian roots in Meteghan River have my deepest gratitude.

Martin Kennelly and Carolyn Passmore, my mentors during my early days at Bell in North Bay, deserve recognition and thanks. Thank you to my friend Catherine Hooper who began the process of nominating me for the Order of Canada and to my many friends on the "A" team of Bell Pioneers who sent in the second nomination. I am certain that helped to expedite the process in my case. From the Bell work centres and garages to the executive boardrooms, I have learned so much. I owe many thanks to all those who touched my life and helped me along the way. My career at Bell shaped who I am today and I am grateful to all of you — you are truly part of my story.

To the many friends I have not mentioned here — you know who you are — I appreciate and treasure your friend-ship. I wanted to name all of you but my editor said, "enough."

Life goes on around you when you put everything else on hold to write a book. Thanks to my "web guy" Roy Gibson who maintains my Web site and managed to keep it current when I was too busy to even think about my business.

To Jack David and the ECW Press team, thank you — from the heart. My book is very different from the books I tried writing in the past. First I tried to write a book about my climb to the VP ranks of Bell. When I was first promoted, the total employee team was in excess of 55,000 and less than 100 of us made up the executive team. It sounded like a book to me. Then I tried to write a book about having battled and beaten cancer, but soon realized there are many books out there about the cancer arena, so why would mine be any different? I checked the availability of different writing courses, but decided an acting course looked like more fun so I signed up for that instead. Finally I knew I had to be serious if I was going to author a book. I made a New Year's resolution to have a book proposal in the hands of at least six publishers by spring 2000. By mid-March my proposal was in the mail. The first rejection came so soon I knew it had not even been read. Not a good start. Then I got some good news: I received an e-mail from Jack David, owner and publisher of ECW: "Thanks for sending your proposal. I think there's a book here, but it's not the one you sent. There are glimpses of your story, but most people are going to want to hear more about you and your mother. I am willing to talk to you about a book that is a more typical memoir/autobiography, possibly written by you, possibly written in conjunction with someone else. Let me know if you'd like to pursue this approach." I called Jack right away, met with him and as they say, the rest is history. An extra special thank you to my editor Jen Hale whose editing skills were tested repeatedly and who continued to say "you're doing a good job" even though I knew better. I could not have picked a better editor to work with and I appreciate your help so very much. To Anjali Kapoor, thank you for your many hours of listening, reading, and writing. Working with you was a pleasure.

To the countless numbers of individuals who gave me

permission to quote from your letters in this book: I apologize if you do not see your words here and I thank you for your support. I worry that you will be disappointed but I hope that you will still allow me to quote from your letters in the future — I have a second book in the dream stage!

To my beloved mother, Mary Rose d'Entremont, thank you for your inspiration. Because of you I have this story to tell. I miss you so much.

Prologue
June 1964

I was eighteen years old and close to graduating from high school the night my mother told me I would have to leave home. The sun was just starting to set as I saw her walking across the lawn from our home to the house next door where I was babysitting. I remember thinking something must be wrong, as Mom never interfered with my babysitting duties.

Judging from the look on her face and the fact that she still had her apron tied around her waist from dinner, I knew she had something serious to talk about. I suddenly felt anxious as my mother sat down across from me, rubbing her hands with worry. She looked at me for a moment, and then launched into what sounded like a well-rehearsed speech.

"This is very difficult for me to say, so please listen carefully. Ask me anything you want when I am finished. I have been saving for one year from our grocery money and have managed to save sixty dollars so that you can move away when you graduate next month."

I stared at her in disbelief. Sixty dollars was a lot of money in 1964 and I wondered how she had managed to save so much. Dad carefully monitored everything that she spent each week. I was more stunned at the thought that I was being "sent away" from home, and I sat there in silence and confusion as she continued to speak.

"I have spoken with your Aunt Edith in North Bay and she would like you to live with them until you find a job and get your own place. I think you should stay with her for at least a year. If you want to come back after one year you can do that, and if you want to move to Toronto or somewhere else you can do that too — but I want you to try this for one year." It seemed I had little choice in the matter, and my thoughts froze when I heard what Mom said next.

"You are doing so well in school and I know you can be a very successful businesswoman — but not in this small town, or even in Halifax. Your father is in all kinds of trouble that you don't even know about. I worry that as Perry Cole's daughter you won't be treated fairly in the business community.

"I want you to make something of the Cole name, but I don't think it will be here."

I was confused by what she was saying about my dad, but Mom had finished what she had come to say. As she got up to leave she looked back at me sitting on the couch, and softly asked if I understood. I told her I did, and did not even consider questioning her judgement. She didn't question whether or not I would succeed at finding a job and starting a career — she had faith I could do it. Mom always instilled confidence in her four daughters and we knew she would do anything she could to help us. I could tell she had made up her mind by the tone in her voice, and once Mom made a decision, there was no looking back.

My mind was racing. I had only been away from my home overnight, but in a month I would be leaving for good. Mom was giving me an opportunity that she had never had herself — the chance to move from a small town that offered so little to a larger city, a good job, and a new life. Although it would be difficult to leave my family and friends, it was time for a clean break if I wanted a career in business.

It was dark when I finished my babysitting job, and I walked back slowly to the house I had lived in for eighteen years. As I entered our home it seemed different now that I knew I would be leaving. I was sad and yet I felt a surge of excitement as I considered how my life was about to change.

Heart of the Valley

In a town the size of Wilmot, there weren't any secrets —
everyone knew everything about everyone else. Small towns
are known for their gossip and general nosiness, and Wilmot
was no exception. In the 1940s and '50s, with a population of
only 600, it was more of a small village than a town. It was
the perfect place for a child to grow up and it was filled with
all sorts of places for us to explore.

Wilmot could have been a replica of any other village in
small town Nova Scotia. Houses lined both sides of the main
road, and the only other buildings were Laurie's Lunch (a
restaurant), and Harnish's convenience store. If you wanted to
do any shopping you had to drive to Middleton, the closest
town. I always thought of Wilmot as being a proud community — people might not have had a lot of money, but they
took pride in their homes and kept them well looked after. I
feel the same way about Wilmot today.

Mom and Dad moved to the area before I was born. Perry Cole and Mary d'Entremont were married in 1942, and moved to an apartment in Middleton that same year; my parents would live in a number of different apartments until they could afford their own home. Lois, my oldest sister, was born the year following their marriage. Dad was a mechanic and later owned a BA service station in Middleton. Mom spent the early years of her marriage making a home and caring for Lois. I was born on March 28, 1946, the same year, I was later told, the Bluenose, Nova Scotia's prize sailing vessel, went down during a squall off a reef in Haiti. Not an auspicious beginning to my life, but one that I did not learn about until years later.

Mom and Dad moved to a home of their own in 1949, when I was three years old and Lois was six. My dad and his brothers built our home and Mom was thrilled to have such a beautiful home to raise "her girls."

I was the baby in the family until Lorraine came along. When she came home from the hospital everyone called her a beautiful baby. No one had ever called me that, and I was immediately jealous of my new sister. The most repeated comment regarding my looks was that I had my father's nose — it was always said in a tone that was less than flattering. It took me at least eight months before I stopped asking my mother how long Lorraine would be living with us and when she would be going back. By the time Connie was born, I had changed my attitude and I was proud to be the big sister; I loved showing off both of my younger siblings.

When I was young our house seemed huge: it was a two-storey, white, clapboard-style house with three very small bedrooms, a dining room, living room, bathroom, kitchen, large porch, and front hallway with a huge staircase on the main floor. The living room with hardwood floors took up one half of the main level, and I always saw it as a beautiful room with the light pouring in from many large windows. At the top of the staircase was a wide landing where we did our homework every night at a big long table. My bedroom was quite small, but it was cozy with a sloped ceiling. Since we each shared a room with one sister there was not much space for more than a bed, a small dresser, and some cubbyholes, which I used to store my collection of marbles. We didn't have a bathroom or running water when we moved in and it wasn't until I was nine years old that we finally had it installed in the house. Of course, most families at the time did not have running water and had an outhouse in the backyard. Ours was a two-hole outhouse, a symbol of stature in the neighbourhood. The White girls next door were jealous that we had a better outhouse than they did — theirs only had one hole. (With a house of four girls it was probably a godsend to my parents that they could send us out there in pairs.) The outhouse was always filled with Eaton's and Simpsons catalogues — for obvious reasons.

Since we didn't even have a well on our property, Dad would carry two buckets of water every morning from our neighbour's well. To this day Lois and I still have very clear memories of having our baths in the kitchen sink. One evening I caused quite a disturbance as I was having my bath. I was playing with my favourite marble — a large robin's egg blue marble — and Mom told me to let Lois have it. She didn't mean permanently, but I misunderstood and decided to swallow it rather than share. The marble lodged in my throat and many anxious moments later we "retrieved" it. My stunt *did* have the desired result, however: Lois didn't want it anymore.

Several years were spent looking for water on our own property and I was very sick of bathing in the kitchen by the time we struck a well. Mom was even more relieved than we were to finally have indoor plumbing. The day the taps started trickling water, Mom made a huge production of opening the front door of the house and heaving the two buckets through the doorway and off the porch. And that is where they stayed for days. We knew it was an important occasion, because Mom rarely made such a big display of her emotions.

The one thing that stood out about our house was the large circular paved driveway at the front of our property — I think it was the only paved driveway in Wilmot. We were also one of the first in the area to have a television set, and it was an exciting time for our whole family. I was six years old when the great event happened and I remember different neighbours traipsing through our house to view this new invention. We watched anything we could during the hours the TV was on — I even found the test pattern enticing. But *The Ed Sullivan Show* was my favourite and I couldn't wait to get to school the next morning to give my friends a recap of who had been on and what they had done.

Despite the lure of the TV, there was plenty to do around Wilmot to fill our days. Our house backed on to a huge meadow, and as kids, my sisters and I and our neighbours would spend countless hours playing with next to nothing but our imagination, especially in the summer. Our next-door neighbours were the Whites and they had one son and four daughters close to our ages. Phyllis White and I were best friends when we were young and we did everything together. Our mothers were also best friends and would spend many afternoons chatting while they waited for us to come home from school. Daisy

White was like a second mother to me, and Phyllis and I would beg her for treats to take to the meadow with us.

Most of my memories of my childhood centre on Phyllis and I figuring out ways to amuse ourselves. One of our favourite things was a game we called Floating Charlies. We would each get a Javex bottle, head down to the river that ran through the meadow, and race the "Charlies." We could spend hours chasing those bottles down the different river paths, yelling and screaming to see who was winning. Or we would wander down to Harnish's convenience store and spend a good half hour carefully considering what we would spend our nickel or penny on — licorice or Jawbreakers. (Phyllis recalls today that I always had the nickel and she had the penny.)

Phyllis's older brother and I made ourselves very ill one day when we drank oil from the top of an oil barrel near our home. We were playing outside, needed a drink of water and our mothers would not give us one. I convinced Georgie that the liquid in the barrel was just water that had collected after a rainstorm so why not drink it? After all, we were thirsty and no one would give us a drink. He reluctantly shared a swallow with me . . . and got just as sick as I did. Being sick was bad enough, then I was punished for "my actions." (I was not totally sure what that meant.)

In the mid '50s we took a trip to the U.S. as a family. We began our drive home after much talk about not mentioning what we had purchased and were bringing back across the border. Dad warned me (it seemed I was the only "talker" they were worried about) that if I said anything at all the nice man at customs would take my play iron that I had purchased with my very own money. When we got there, everything was going very well — the man liked all of us and was asking Dad how he and Mom happened to have four such beautiful daughters. I liked this guy! Finally, the big question: "Have you anything to declare?"

"Nothing at all," said my dad. Then, I believe he decided maybe he should add something so he said, "Well actually sir, Carol has a kid's play iron in the back seat, but that's about it." My mind started to spin. Without hesitation I shouted, "Yeah, and my dad is wearing two pairs of pants, my mom has a sweater under her seat and every single one of my sisters got something too!" If I was going to be in trouble I wanted company. The customs officer laughed out loud and said, "Off you go, and try to keep that one quiet in the future."

When Lorraine and Connie were very small, Mom would make Lois and me take them with us everywhere we went, and we thought it was such a nuisance. We would try to exclude Connie and Lorraine from anything we did, usually because we thought they were still too young. We had the typical fights that four sisters living in a house together would have — the younger girls would play with my marbles or someone might be in the bathroom too long. When I was nine Lois and I caught jaundice, and both of us were stuck at home for what seemed like an eternity. The monotony of being sick was broken by a surprise from our Aunt Edith, who sent us one gift to open daily for the entire month we were ill. I recovered quickly but Lois developed rheumatic fever and was very ill. She was in bed for ten months, missed more than a year of school, and when she did return to school she was so weak she could only attend morning classes. I paid little attention to her health, but I didn't think it was all that fair that she didn't have to stay in school all day. There was entirely too much attention being paid to "poor little Lois" for my liking!

Lois and I shared a large wooden dollhouse when we were very small, albeit as she would tell the story, I didn't like sharing that, either. Mom solved the problem by telling us that one week the dollhouse was mine to play with and the next week it belonged to Lois. During the week Lois was in control I would get up in my sleep and move all the doll furniture back to the way I liked it. Lois was never convinced that I was really walking in my sleep.

My sisters and I spent a great deal of our childhood playing with each other, but we were also just as happy to play with our other friends and cousins in the neighbourhood. I loved the freedom of being able to stay outside for hours. During the summer Mom would allow us to walk by ourselves to my grandmother's farm for an afternoon — this was a big deal because it was a very long walk. Dad grew up with many siblings on the Cole farm, just outside of Wilmot. On warm sunny days, Phyllis and I would walk up the long dirt road, picking berries en route to Grammy's house. Walking into the farmyard at Grammy's was like entering another world. There were cows, horses, sheep, and pigs. Someone was always rushing around doing chores. It was a place where you were allowed to get dirty, and it was heaven for us. We would sometimes help gather eggs from the dozens of hens that were always a fixture in the front yard. I walked around in wide-eyed wonder since there was so much going on and so many people helping out.

My memories of Grammy herself involve the kitchen, not the farmyard. There was baking going on at the house at any time of day, and Grammy made everything in great quantities. Pies, bread, biscuits, and cookies were always coming out of the oven. Grammy would stand amidst all the chaos, surrounded by huge bags of flour, baking away. I couldn't imagine how anyone could put together that much food. On holidays, like Christmas, we would go there and a table would be set up the length of the house to hold all the food for dinner — and all the Coles.

Many Sundays our family would go to Grammy's and we would end up playing outside with our cousins. We saw my dad's family quite often growing up, and my mother would sit and talk with our aunts while the children played outside. I loved my Auntie Marie and she always gave great presents. Auntie Marie seemed to sense that I was not getting along well with my dad and she would often seek me out to ask how "things were going" in my life — although we did not talk about anything specific. I appreciated this even as a very young child, especially since she was Dad's sister and I thought she treated me in a special way when we had these talks at Grammy's house. My uncles would chase me and tell me they were going to rub butter on my nose to make it grow bigger. That always upset me, but they acted this way with all of us so I knew they weren't really making fun of my nose.

Mom had grown up in Meteghan River, a French community in Nova Scotia where everyone spoke Acadian French. Sadly we drove there only once a year to visit my mother's family, and always during the summer. We loved the dulse and dried fish. It was a big family event and at the time I didn't find it odd that Mom only got to visit her own family once a year. That's the way it was with anyone who married into the Cole family — they became a Cole and not only lost their name, but their identity as well. To try to keep her background alive, my mother would teach us a bit of Acadian French and we tried to practise it at the supper table by saying "Pass the salt" or "Pass the bread" in the other language. Dad would make fun of us, saying the language sounded strange, and so the tradition didn't last.

Dad wasn't really involved in our moral or ethical upbringing — that was Mom's job. She was the one who instilled order in the house, whether it was teaching us how to cook or clean up after ourselves. Every Saturday morning Lois and I had to be awake by 9 a.m. to do our own ironing for the week. Mom would wash clothes in a huge wringer washing machine and then she would hang them on the line to dry. By the time we got up everything would be ready for ironing and Mom would always supervise. Even though Mom always had so many things to do on weekend mornings, I always felt this ironing time was my special time with her. She made an effort to know what was going on in my life. Whether we talked about school, boyfriends, or my dreams for the future, Mom had a story to tell or some sound advice to pass on. She was one of those mothers who just sensed things. She always had a way of checking up on us when we were doing our homework to make sure it was getting done.

Mom also guided our religious upbringing and we never missed church on Sunday unless we were very ill. And if we felt too sick to attend church, Mom would make sure we stayed in the house for the rest of the weekend until school on Monday. So there wasn't much of a choice — church or house arrest for the weekend. Mom was extremely strict about arriving at the church early. We would be there at 10 a.m. for an 11 a.m. mass, and we waited at the back for the early mass to end. My sisters and I would always complain about it, but I believe Mom liked her time alone to think. Dad did not attend mass with us, but it was his job to drive us to and from church every Sunday. We also went to Sunday school and summer school at St. Monica's, where we learned about Communion and Confession. I had my first argument with Mom concerning my "sins" when I was nine years old. Every Saturday evening Mom would review our sins with each of us before we went to confession on Sunday. It always amazed me how she knew exactly what we had done during the week that was sinful. I really liked the idea of confession — three Hail Marys and you are forgiven and can start the week with a clean slate! That particular week she reminded me I had told three little lies, yelled at my sisters for no reason, and swore numerous times. I argued with Mom that I had sworn with permission, so it couldn't be a sin. One of Dad's friends at the garage had taught me a funny saying so I could remember his name — Charlie. He encouraged me to memorize this saying: "Charlie hump back, kiss my ass, and jump back." I thought it was the funniest thing I had ever heard and repeated it to anyone who would listen, including Mom. Now she was making sure I shared it with the priest as well — as usual Mom was always one step ahead of me. I don't recall the priest laughing.

While Mom was raising her girls, Dad spent most of his time at the service station in Middleton and hanging out with his buddies at the air force base. My dad's reputation was probably already set by the time I was born and growing up in Wilmot; I was five years old when I realized people looked at him a little differently. One day when I was at the garage I heard some men talking about my dad and someone called him an outcast. At first I thought they just meant he was sitting outside, and for a time after that when people would call or come to the house asking for my father I would say, "He must be outcast." I didn't understand it was wrong, until my mother heard me and explained that if I didn't know what the word meant I was not to use it. Most of the trouble in our lives at the time related to my father's drinking, not paying his bills on time, and the fact that his temper had gotten the better of him on too many occasions. My mother tried to keep us pretty sheltered from the rumours, but on occasion we would hear a whisper and know something was not quite right.

My relationship with my dad was always different from the one he had with my sisters. My father never saw me as one of his girls — my sisters were the girls and I was always Carol, not Carol Ann. I was seven years old when Connie was born, and I remember Dad being very sad when he was told we had a new sister. He became quiet and sat drinking his beer after he had heard the news, probably resigning himself to the fact he would never have a son. In some ways I might have been the son he wanted and as a result he treated me differently. When we went camping as a family he would say, "Mommy, you and the girls make dinner and Carol and I will pitch the tents." I think he saw me as being tougher than my sisters, and treated me accordingly. There was also a side of me that I think he resented — it might have been because I was very confrontational with him.

I had my first beating from Dad when I was six years old. As our neighbours Brad and Bea passed our house in their horse and buggy Lois called out to them. They replied, "Good morning, Lois" so I tried the same thing but got no response. I spoke louder but got no response. I shouted and got no response. I swore at them and got a response — from Dad. It was to be the first of several beatings, though he never touched my sisters or my mother. I always seemed to do something to provoke his temper, even when I wasn't trying to. One Sunday morning I was playing with my huge marble collection when

I accidentally dropped some near the stair landing. As each one clattered down the wooden stairs, it woke everyone up and Dad yelled from the bedroom, "One more peep out of you and I'll whip you until the blood runs out of your ass." As I scrambled to pick them up, one dropped out of my hand and the sound echoed throughout the house as it bounced down each stair. Dad got out of bed and gave me such a beating that I was unable to go to mass that morning.

It was hard to accept that Dad treated me differently, but I found refuge in other activities away from home, where I could be myself. Even though I wasn't an ace student at school, I loved learning about different places and people. In Grade Three I thought I had found *the* woman who would be my hero. Her name was Gloria Sandfree. I didn't know much about her except that we sang a song in her honour every day in class. She must have done some wonderful things and I couldn't wait to learn who she was. Imagine my disappointment when I realized the woman I was singing about didn't even exist. I had mistaken the words in "O Canada," and should have been singing "O Canada, glorious and free" — *not* my version of "O Canada, Gloria Sandfree."

When I was ten years old and in Grade Five, I developed a stuttering problem that was so bad I could not even finish a sentence sometimes. I think it was probably caused by all the anxiety and insecurity I felt with my father. He would yell at me at the dinner table and say things like, "Your little sisters can speak better than you can." One evening my mother sat down with me and we talked about finding a way to solve my problem. She suggested I should speak with my teacher and see if she could help me. Mom felt that if I was able to talk it through, I might feel better at school and she was right.

The next day I approached my teacher and she began to coach me in reading aloud to the class. I became determined to find a way to cure my "problem" and I worked at it until I was comfortable enough to recite a poem at my Grade Five graduation. It actually worked, and I eventually began to enter public speaking contests, even winning one! My talk was entitled "Childhood Memories" and I spoke about having met Princess Margaret when she made a train trip through Middleton. Mom made me a blue skirt from a new fabric called "crushed ice" and bought me a sixty-yard crinoline for the competition. The crinoline was bigger than I was! I felt both beautiful and confident. Mom was so proud of me and would attend every public speaking event — I would see her in the audience and my confidence would grow. This was the first time I realized that if I put my mind to something, it could be accomplished. Little did I know that conquering my fear of public speaking would evolve into a career later in life.

I used this new confident attitude when it was time to transfer to the high school in Middleton after grade school. It was a big change since I now had to take the bus, and all the new people who attended the huge school overwhelmed me. As the bus left Wilmot and entered Middleton I would watch for the red-heart-shaped sign boldly saying "Middleton — Heart of the Valley." I watched for that sign every day and loved it! Although I found my classes interesting, it was my extra-curricular activities that provided me with a new love: sports. My gym teacher, Mr. Peppard, was an integral part in cultivating my determination to be a first-rate athlete. I tried out for every sport, but it seemed something was always holding me back: I was fast but not fast enough, tall but not tall enough, strong but not strong enough. Yet it was Mr. Peppard who convinced me that if I put my mind to it, I could be the best at anything, and not just sports. Mr. Peppard was my first true mentor and to this day I continue to seek his advice whenever I'm in Middleton.

High school was so much more fun than the two-room schoolhouse I had gone to in Wilmot. I tried to be involved in everything so I could meet new people. I was still best friends with Phyllis and in high school I met another girl who became a life-long friend, Donna Cross. Donna had moved to Middleton the year we were both in Grade Ten, and I was a little in awe of the new girl. She had flawless skin, a beautiful face, and a grown-up figure at sixteen years of age. Beside her I was a skinny, flat-chested girl whose broad shoulders were a source of constant discontent. One day I was sitting at Laurie's Lunch counter having a soda and admiring the ring I had just been given by my first steady boyfriend, Jerry Adams. In walked Donna and plunked herself down beside me at the counter. We had not actually spoken until this point, and when she asked me if the ring on my hand was from Jerry Adams, I proudly said yes. I asked her how she knew it was Jerry's ring, and her reply was, "Oh I just gave it back to him."

We stared at each other for a moment and then burst out laughing — the more we talked the more we liked each other. From that first meeting we went on to become best friends. Donna was there to sympathize with me when Jerry Adams dumped me a few months later. Mom comforted me as much as Donna did, telling me that it was hard to get over your first boyfriend. And although I dated other guys during the rest of my high school years, I was never interested in anyone the way I was with Jerry.

Mastering "the twist" was on my list of things to do as a teenager. Each night after supper I would go next door and

Barb Beals and I would watch and learn from Barb's older sister Diane. I thought Diane was absolutely the best dancer in the world. Later, their mother Marguerite would marry my Uncle Carmen and we would all be related, but at the time Barb and I were simply teenagers learning to dance. Their apartment had a very long hall and we would twist up and down that hall for hours. Marguerite would laugh and encourage us to "dance like Diane." My problem, it seemed, was my hips — or lack thereof.

Mom was my confidante throughout my high school years and we would talk every day when I got home from school. She helped Donna and I through our many dates with boys and was always there to lend a comforting shoulder to cry on. I remember sitting in our family car with Donna the day she broke up with her sweetheart Randy. It was raining heavily and we were listening to romantic songs on the radio. Donna was crying. Even though Mom wasn't in the car she had sensed somehow that something was wrong. She brought us a snack on a tray to cheer us up. Mom was always in tune with what we were feeling.

Many of my talks with Mom after school were filled with gossip or lengthy recaps of my basketball tournaments or track and field events. She loved to know what was going on, and I held nothing back. In my last year of high school, Mom would sometimes steer our conversations to what I would do after graduation. She had a way of inquiring that didn't sound pushy, but I knew she was thinking about my future. My friends and I had always talked about what we would be doing after graduation and most of us just assumed we would move to the big city of Halifax and get a job. Out of my graduating class of eighty people, a few would be going to university, but for most of my girlfriends, getting a job in Halifax was a priority. Several also had steady boyfriends and many were already planning to get married in the next couple of years. In a small town a measure of success is your husband, your children, and your home — your career or job is always secondary. I knew it would be different for me.

University was not an option for me because of the cost and in all honesty, I wasn't interested in university at that time. In my last year of high school I had switched to a general commercial program that taught me the "skills of the secretarial world," which was clearly where I was headed. I was determined to have a "career" and I think my mother recognized that ambition from our many discussions. I was always interested in business, but at eighteen that interest was an uninformed one. I may not have understood how a business worked, but I was fascinated with what was going on in the business world.

One of the discussions I would have with my mother centred on the difference between a job and a career. If I typed forever as a secretary it would be a job, but if I *supervised* the girls who were typing, I would have a career. I talked about so many different things I would like to do, and Mom would punctuate the conversation with the question, "Is that a job or a career?" I knew she was encouraging me, and I know she was very thankful that I would have an opportunity to become successful.

When Mom offered me the chance to move to North Bay and find a job, I knew she had listened to all our conversations carefully. She had been planning for more than a year, and had seen how different my priorities were from my other friends. She knew I didn't have any thoughts at all about marriage, kids, or settling down in one place. It took me a while to understand why Mom was so adamant about me leaving my home and finding a job in North Bay; up until then, I had taken my relationship with my mother for granted because she was always there for me. Now she was encouraging me to leave the security of a place I had always known to pursue my dreams. I'm sure she didn't want me to go, yet she knew it was the only avenue available at the time.

The first person I told was Donna. She was very surprised that my mom was allowing me to leave. When I told everyone else at school, they began speculating about how much more money I could make. One girl told me she had heard you could make sixty-five dollars a week in Ontario; I figured if I could make five more dollars a week than my mother had taken a year to save, then it was worth it to leave. My last few weeks of school sped by as I spent every spare moment thinking about my upcoming move. Like Mom, once the decision was made, I did not look back.

The only problem was my father. Mom had told Dad about her plans for me and a couple of days later she told me he was not happy with the news. The day he decided to drive me home from his gas station himself, instead of getting someone else at the garage to do it, I knew we were about to have a talk.

"This is damn foolishness," was the first thing he said during the drive. My father was never a man of many words when he had to get something out.

"You mean me going to North Bay?" I asked.

"There's no need of it and I'm not giving you any money, either. You're not going to North Bay."

I knew if I told Dad about the money Mom had saved she would get in trouble, so I simply said, "Well I'm going and I wrote a letter to Aunt Edith and she has told me I can stay there." Dad was upset when he heard this because Aunt Edith was his sister, and he felt Mom had gone behind his back to send me to North Bay. That was the end of the discussion for him.

All I could think about was getting to Halifax and boarding that train for North Bay. I was excited about the chance to live with Aunt Edith, whom I had always considered my favourite aunt. When I got home I said to Mom, "Dad was upset. Do you think he will drive me to Halifax?" Mom told me not to worry and that the whole family would be going to see me off. When I think about it today, I'm sure that he made life even more difficult for Mom around that period of time. And it made me more aggressive with him. Although Mom had tried to keep it from us, I had heard rumblings about the financial troubles we were in. I knew Dad's business was not doing well, and Mom had hinted that he wasn't even paying our phone bill. Before I left I confronted him about the phone being disconnected.

"So I understand we aren't even going to have a telephone," I said in a very flippant tone.

He just looked at me and said, "Your mother put that notion in your mind, and it's not true." By this time, I felt that if I could give as good as I would get with my father in terms of confronting him, at some point he would see me as an equal. But that did not happen before I left and it still hasn't happened today as an adult. I wanted some sort of acknowledgement that he was proud of the fact I was graduating and was going to have a career. The closest he ever came to showing me affection before I left was on graduation night at the high school. As I walked past him and my family after receiving my diploma, he reached out his hand and messed up my hair. I remember feeling a swell of pride that he had shown his approval through such a public display of affection. (I tried to ignore the smell of liquor on his breath.)

My oldest sister, Lois, was the most excited for me that I was leaving. She had recently married and was living in Halifax, expecting her first child. She had her own life and saw this as a unique opportunity for me. My two younger sisters, Connie and Lorraine, were more excited about getting their own bedrooms than concerned with me leaving.

There was little fanfare the night before I left for North Bay. I had spent the day packing my one suitcase for the trip, though I didn't have much to take. I even had to borrow the suitcase from an aunt, since our family rarely travelled anywhere. As an eighteen-year-old girl, most of my preparations were pretty superficial. I didn't have a lot of clothing and everything that I did have fit in the one suitcase. I was at the point in my life where I was extremely self-conscious about being skinny so I took the only clothes that made me look like I had hips. Inverted pleats were all the rage at the time, and I had two skirts — one in green and one in blue. They were heavier winter skirts, but I knew I would be able to afford a whole new wardrobe on sixty-five dollars a week and very few expenses in North Bay. The rest of my clothes I would be wearing on the trip, so I filled my suitcase with a few other personal possessions. I took a couple of "special" marbles, saved from my big marble collection. I walked away from everything and everyone I knew with that suitcase and a plan — I was going to start all over again. I also took three pictures, without frames: one of Mom; one of the whole family; and one of Lorraine, Connie, and I. My mom made me put the pictures in my purse so I could look at them on the train — although I couldn't imagine I would start missing my family that soon.

Dad wasn't home for dinner the night before I left, and it was a typical evening. Mom, Connie, Lorraine, and I had dinner and talked about the trip to Halifax and who was going to come with us. All my friends wanted to see me off at the train station and were talking about whether they would follow us into the city in their car or meet us at the train station. I was a little nervous about the two-day train trip to North Bay. Mom didn't want me travelling alone and had arranged for me to take the trip with my Aunt Margaret and her two children, Susan and Larry. Since Aunt Margaret was on her way to North Bay for a vacation, she was happy to take me along, and arranged to meet me the next day at the station. I was also anxious to finish supper so I could get on the phone and talk to Donna about the next day. Between Donna and I we had it all worked out — what I would wear the first day of work (even though I didn't know where that was going to be), how tightly I would curl my hair — some of the most important things for a girl my age!

Dad still wasn't home by the time I went to bed, and I thought Mom and I might talk about my leaving, but we didn't. That was very much like Mom — we had said what needed to be said and now it was time to make it happen. She had noticed me talking to Connie and Lorraine earlier in the evening as I tried to explain my trip and she had not joined the conversation. She had a sad look on her face but she kept busy ironing clothes, setting the table for breakfast the next morning, and, I am sure, wondering what shape Dad would be in when he came home that night. He had started to drink more and I know it worried Mom. As I said goodnight to my two small sisters I felt a twinge of loneliness beginning to set in. Eventually I closed my suitcase for the final time and went to bed.

The next day was sunny and bright, a typical spring day in Nova Scotia. I still have the photograph Lorraine took of me on the front steps of our house as everyone packed the car for the trip. The photo shows a nervous young woman, standing awkwardly on the steps clutching her purse. I was determined to look good, even though I would be wearing the same clothes for two days on the train. That morning I had dressed carefully in my only good "shift" dress, my one pair of white high-heeled shoes, a coat, and a purse, borrowed from my mother at the last minute. My friends piled into one car, and with my family in the other we started on the two-hour trip to Halifax. It wasn't a pleasant ride, since Dad was blaming Mom for the sombre mood in the car. You could tell by the abrupt way he talked to her that he was only going along with things because the train ticket had already been bought. When we got to the train station in Halifax, Mom handed me the one-way train ticket to North Bay and sixty dollars in cash, telling me to put it in my purse. My friends met us on the platform and we waited for the train.

By now I was really angry with Dad for the silent treatment he had given Mom on the way in. So when he pulled out a big roll of money from his pocket and said "Carol, how much do you want?" my reply was one that I regret even today. I looked at him defiantly and said, "I don't need any money, Dad. Mom's given me all the money I need."

Dad slowly turned to Mom and said, "We'll talk about that."

I was trying to brag about what Mom had done for me in front of my friends, who all knew that Dad was the one who usually gave out the money. Everybody outside of the family loved my father for his "generosity." If I went bowling with my friends, he would insist on telling me in front of them to treat everyone to a game. Or he would give the high school sports teams cars to drive to out-of-town games, and never let the high school administration pay for gas. Dad treated everyone differently than he treated his own family — and money was always out of our reach. So I knew my moment of bragging would cause my mother a great deal of heartache later since she was the one who had to ride home with him in the car. Immediately the excitement of the upcoming train ride was over for me and once again the focus was on money.

My mom started crying and I hugged her goodbye first. I was amazed even then, she never once said, "I hope I haven't made a mistake." In her heart, she knew this was the right thing to do, and the only way for me to begin my career in the business world. I turned to Lorraine and Connie and gathered them in my arms — they seemed so small. Lorraine said in her most grown-up voice, "We'll write to you all the time," and Connie chimed in with, "Yes, Mom says we have to."

And then I was in the midst of my friends, going around and hugging them goodbye. Donna was trying to make jokes, promising to write and telling me we would get together as soon as I came home for a visit. I hugged my mom once more and then got on the train. I found my seat close to Aunt Margaret and her kids, then sat back and cried for the longest time. I felt overwhelmed, very young, and alone.

While I was sniffling away, a cute air force guy came along, sat down across from me and asked me why I was crying. I said I was leaving home and he asked me if it was my first time away from home. I nodded tearfully. He told me he was going to Camp Borden and that leaving home was a good thing for him. We chatted for a while and he asked me if he could buy me a drink. I was quick to say I didn't drink and he changed his tactic. "How about a walk then? We can talk while we are walking and maybe by the time we get to the club car you will be ready for your first drink."

I refused again and he became frustrated with me. He reached into his pocket, pulled out a dime (which was the price of placing a call at a pay phone at the time), threw it at me and said, "Give me a call when you grow up." Then he walked away. But instead of being offended, I found this very funny and turned to my aunt with a smile, saying, "Mom was right, things are looking up already. I've made ten cents, and we're not even there yet."

Broad Shoulders

*E*veryone has a favourite relative in their life; someone with whom they form a special bond. For me, that was my Aunt Edith. I remember her visits to Wilmot every summer. She would take an avid interest in all of us and spend afternoons chatting with my mother. Mom had spoken to her the previous summer about allowing me to come to North Bay, and I now realized they had spent the entire year planning my future.

Aunt Edith, Uncle Ken, and their sons Chuck, Brian, and Gary met me at the train and took me back to their house. I instantly fell in love with the room she had prepared for my stay. She had obviously worked very hard to make my room feminine and inviting, from the curtains on the window to the handmade pillows and bedspread. As she helped me unpack, Aunt Edith asked if I had brought any pictures with me. When I took the photos my mom had given me out of my purse, she said her first gift to me would be frames for each of the pictures. She was anxious that I make the room my own so I wouldn't feel too homesick.

In my mind Aunt Edith represented that "career woman" I wanted to be: she was a salesperson at a local shoe store in North Bay, she had her own hairdressing business in her home, and she was a well-known seamstress. My Uncle Ken worked for Ontario Hydro and spent a great deal of time away from his family. The very idea that she kept three jobs going while looking after her boys was astounding to me. I admired her so much and it seemed natural that she would be the one who would help me find a job.

Living at my aunt and uncle's house was very different from what I was used to at home. The family seemed financially more stable than my own and there was an open exchange of money within the household. This was something really new to me — my dad had always held the purse strings in our family and my mother was never allowed money of her own. Before leaving home Mom had talked to me about the importance of paying for my room and board as soon as I arrived, so I broached the subject with my aunt before I finished unpacking. We agreed that twelve dollars a week was a fair amount and I immediately handed over the money from the sixty dollars my mother had given me. Even though my aunt wanted me to wait until I had a job, I felt it part of my duty to pay my way. Over the course of each week, Aunt Edith always tried to give me that twelve dollars back in some way. She would give me two dollars to go to the store to buy milk and not ask for the change. Or, she would make me several outfits for work and never ask for money for the material. I know she enjoyed doing my hair and making new clothes for me, which was very different than dressing her three sons.

Aunt Edith did things to show that she was excited to have me there and that I was part of their family. She treated me like a daughter, helping me start a career and showing concern for my health and upbringing. She told me that she had booked a dentist appointment for me the next day and that she would pay for the first few appointments until I could pay her back. I immediately felt a warm rush of gratitude for this woman who understood what was important to me. I had written Aunt Edith the moment I found out I would be moving to North Bay to ask her to call the dentist, because even before finding a job, my goal was to finally have something done about my teeth.

Ever since I was a small child, I remember having insecurities about my teeth. There were spaces between them and they were crooked. Growing up, I went to a dentist a number of times and then, with the bills unpaid, the dentist finally refused to see me. Mom explained to me that we would have to cope without a dentist until Dad paid the bills. Dad had dentures and didn't believe the rest of the family needed to see a dentist, so that was that. When I was eleven years old, I developed a very bad abscess and Mom insisted Dad take me to a dentist in town, so he finally did. But we didn't go to our regular dentist. I knew something was wrong when we climbed up the fire escape on the side of the building to see the "dentist." He froze my gums and began to pull a tooth out. I suspect it was the large abscess that prevented the freezing from working, and soon the pain was so overwhelming I fainted. It was a horrifying experience, and I hated sharing it with Mom when I arrived home. I felt totally helpless about my teeth. When I was in Grade Seven, I decided I would take matters into my own hands and I visited the local dentist on the way home from school. I politely asked him if he would fix my teeth in exchange for babysitting his children or cleaning his house. He refused and I was devastated. He explained that he would be happy to have me as a client if my father would first pay all the outstanding bills he had on file. I walked home slowly and cried as I told Mom what I had tried to do. She cried too.

Edith realized how important it was for me to see a dentist right away and she accompanied me to my dentist appointment. It was obvious I had some serious problems with my teeth, and as soon as I opened my mouth the dentist took one look and asked, "How could you let your teeth go like this?" My aunt gave him a searing look and literally shouted, "Let me tell you about my brother, who happens to be this young girl's father!" By the time she finished her tirade, the poor man was almost crying. He quickly made appointments to see me every day before I started my new job to try and fix my teeth. Each day as I would leave his office I would feel more and more confident and by the time I started working I was able to laugh and smile without holding my hand over my mouth, something I'd done for most of my life. Aunt Edith had given me such a wonderful gift with her support. She had not only listened — she had understood.

I learned so many things from Aunt Edith. She loved dressing me in new fashionable clothes. She made me my first sleeveless dress before I started work, and even convinced me that the arms I thought were too thin were just fine. She shared with me in a whisper that she knew I was walking around with my arms pressed to each side of my body to make them look fatter (I thought I had the world fooled!). I didn't see Aunt Edith as a mother figure, but more as a big sister or protector.

She knew who was hiring in the town, and because she was a well-known member of the community, having her as my reference helped me find a job. She told me that the Bank of Nova Scotia and Bell Canada were hiring and I immediately filled out applications for both. When I returned home, I jokingly asked if anyone had called. She told me that indeed someone had. Bill Stevenson, from the Bank of Nova Scotia, had phoned just after I had filled out the application form to arrange for an interview the next day. The position was second stenographer. Look out business world — here I come!

In the morning I was a nervous wreck as I walked to the bank. As part of the interview, Mr. Stevenson dictated a letter to me that was filled with language I could barely understand. I sat frantically for a few moments wondering what I should do. I certainly couldn't type up the letter. The first stenographer, Judy, came over and introduced herself. She knew I was in trouble, and asked where I was from. When I said Nova Scotia she told me Mr. Stevenson was also a Maritimer. She then went and spoke to him, and a minute later as I sat staring at the blank piece of paper, Mr. Stevenson said he had changed his mind and wanted to dictate another letter to me. This one had to do with a fishing trip back home; I aced it with flying colours. I was offered the job at fifty dollars a week and raced home to share the good news with my aunt. Although the money was a bit less than I had expected from the rich province of Ontario, it was still far better than what I would have made in Halifax.

The following week, after settling into my first job, Bell called me for an interview. I already felt a sense of loyalty to the bank and advised Bell I had found another job that would give me two weeks of vacation at the end of the year. By this time I was feeling homesick and all I could think about was going home in eleven months. I tried to make Bell understand that even though I had just started this job, my first vacation was so important I just couldn't change jobs yet. I had decided to stay in North Bay for Christmas that year. Rather than spend my money on an airline ticket, I bought presents for my whole family. As the holidays approached, I observed everyone at the bank getting ready to go home. Although I was going to be with my aunt and her family, I felt extremely sad when I wrote my mother telling her I wouldn't be there for Christmas. I hadn't spoken with my mother since August 27, the day Lois's first child, Natalie, was born. Mom had asked the phone company to keep the phone connected until the baby was born, and they had agreed, but the next day they cut us off, just as Mom had predicted they would. My only solace was the long letters I wrote to Mom, my sisters, and my friends.

Communicating by letter allowed me to feel like I was having an ongoing conversation with all the people who were important to me. My friend Donna and I wrote to each other every day of the week when I first arrived in North Bay. I am sure the mailman wondered what was in all the letters he delivered to my aunt's house daily. He once commented to her that mail delivery to her address had increased so much his back was hurting.

When Christmas Day finally arrived, I spent the morning crying and missing my family. Everyone had included a personal note with each of the presents they had sent to me, and the distance between us seemed greater that day. I was thankful for my aunt's effort to try to make the holidays as pleasant for me as possible. And I took some solace in the fact that I would be going home for vacation in only six months.

Soon after Christmas, Bell called me again to offer me

another interview. This time I boldly informed them I was *definitely* not interested since I was going home on vacation to see my family in the summer. I didn't give Bell another thought. I spent the next couple of months planning with Donna what I would do during my vacation. We decided we would go to the Teen Town dance the first Saturday night I was home. Donna organized all of our friends and she even arranged for someone to pick me up at my house, since she knew I wouldn't have a phone to call anyone. By the time May ended, Donna had planned every detail of my upcoming vacation. I'll never forget the feeling of landing in Halifax on a sunny day in June after being away from home for almost a year. It is the same sensation that I still enjoy today: home is when I touch down at the airport in Halifax.

I knew something was wrong the moment I walked into our house in Wilmot. My mother was thrilled to see me and made a big fuss about me being home, but she soon revealed that they were going to lose our house. Even worse was the fact my father's job wasn't going to last much longer. Mom and I had a long talk as she told me about all the things that she didn't want to include in her weekly letters. She really opened up to me, and filled me in on so many things — so many sad things. In the past year Dad had taken out a second mortgage on the house in Mom's name. I couldn't understand how this was possible, as Mom had never signed any mortgage papers. She asked me to help her find out how that happened. I felt very mature as Mom discussed the situation with me, and I told her I could "fix it" — after all I *was* working in a bank! She was skeptical and concerned about what I might do, but I was confident that I could solve the problem. I walked straight to the bank that very day to talk to the manager. At the time I thought I had some clout; I explained to him that I knew there was a mortgage on our home in my mom's name and that she had not signed any papers. I then made the mistake of telling him that I too worked in a bank and knew how things worked. I demanded to know who had drawn up the mortgage papers in his bank and wondered out loud if something illegal was going on.

The manager just looked at me in total disbelief and asked, "Does your father know you are here?"

"He doesn't know I'm here and I would prefer that he not know," I boldly replied.

"Well, this is none of your business," he said. "Your father is a good man and a good businessman and he's a friend of mine — now get out of here."

I turned to leave, astounded that my father had so many people fooled. When I returned home I told Mom what I had done. She knew I had gone too far and began telling me Dad would be angry with both of us.

At that moment my father walked through the door — the bank manager had called him immediately. Mom and I were standing in the living room, and I saw him coming towards me. He slapped me so hard on my face that I fell to the floor. He was livid beyond belief and very drunk as he yelled at me.

"So you think you're a big shot now, huh? You leave here and get a job in Ontario and now you think you can talk to my bank manager? There is nothing wrong, we are not going to lose the house, and your mother once again put that idea into your head."

Mom helped me get up. Dad was still shouting about how I should never have bothered to come home as he stormed out of the house. I felt an intense stab of guilt for getting my mother into trouble once again. Mom was doing her very best to keep everything together and here I was making it worse moments after arriving. She quietly told me not to worry, that things would work out. She knew her future was uncertain, but she would deal with that, as she had dealt with everything so far. In the meantime, she wanted my visit to be enjoyable and tried to cheer me up before my sisters came home from school.

During my two-week visit, Dad never once came home at mealtime. It was always Mom, Lorraine, Connie, and I at the table, although Dad sometimes showed up very inebriated at the end of dinner. Despite the dark shadow of Dad's state, I was determined to still enjoy my visit home. The first Saturday night Jimmy Taylor picked me up to go to the Teen Town dance at the high school. Jimmy was a good friend and an excellent dancer, so I was thrilled to be going to the dance with him. Although I had been away for a year, I still knew about everything that was going on in all my friends' lives because Donna's letters had kept me up to date. I remember that whole time being bittersweet as well. I was excited and happy to be out with my friends, but I was also pretty embarrassed about what was happening at home with Dad. Being away from home made the situation seem so much worse to come home to. I was only home for a limited period of time, but it was enough to show me that Dad was now drinking all the time and barely supporting the family.

I spent as much time with Mom as I could during that visit. She was always reassuring me how great it was for her and my sisters to have me home. I had brought my sisters little gifts of stationery and chocolate, but it seemed insignificant compared to everything that I now had. Considering I left home with only a few clothes in a suitcase, I now had more clothes than both of my younger sisters put together. Mom was barely surviving and doing the best she could with what she had. I started to worry about what would happen to Mom and my little sisters, and it terrified me to think she may have to find work outside of the home one day. What would she do, considering she'd been a homemaker all her life? For the first time I thought about how I should help my family financially. I wondered if a job at Bell might include a better salary and the possibility of a career somewhere in my future. Maybe I should not have turned down those interviews, I thought.

It was very hard for me to leave my mom and sisters when my vacation was over. I took a last look around the house I had grown up in, praying that it would still belong to us when I came home for Christmas later that same year. Our house was *our* house and I felt very strongly about that.

I arrived back in North Bay to some very encouraging news. Aunt Edith told me Bell had called again in my absence and she had set up an interview for the following morning. She was going to call the bank and tell them I was sick while I went to the interview. Aunt Edith had always thought Bell would be a better place for me career-wise. We had already had many discussions about how very few women seemed to be in a position of power at the bank. That reasoning, combined with my family's precarious financial situation, prompted me to give serious consideration to making a job change. I arrived at my interview the next morning determined to get the job of service order typist for Bell.

The first person I met at the North Bay business office of Bell Canada was a supervisor named Carolyn Passmore. She gave me a tour of the building and showed me the large teletype machine I would be operating if I were successful in getting the job. When Carolyn asked if I had any questions I said no, but that I was anxious to meet the manager, Mr. Kennelly. I suggested that if he was going to make a decision about hiring me I should spend some time with him. I had made the assumption that this decision would be his to make. I didn't realize that Mr. Kennelly was already ahead of his time — he allowed his supervisors to make those decisions! I met him, we talked for a few minutes, and he then turned to Carolyn and said "So, what do you think? Should we hire her?" I had already been conditioned to think the men made all the decisions in business. Luckily, she didn't take any offense and she gave me the job. And, it paid seven dollars more per week than I was making at the bank. At the time, I had no idea how much guidance I would receive from Carolyn Passmore during my career.

My aunt was proud of me. She knew this job would be the beginning of my career. Those were the words I wanted to hear, and the reason I had come to North Bay. I knew that I was not going to be a service order typist for long; I was happy to start there and was proud of my "big job at the Bell," as I would call it, but there would be bigger jobs. I knew it.

Just after starting at Bell I went to Hamilton for my typing course. A hotel room *and* expense account — wow! My uncle Andy, Mom's brother, lived in Hamilton and he took me to dinner several times. It was wonderful to hear his stories about Mom and her siblings. I was a great Hamilton Tiger-Cat football fan and he knew where the team hung out, so we followed them around. He was living a faster life than I had known and I enjoyed seeing the world through his eyes. When I completed my typing course and returned to the office, I put everything into my job. When I had nothing to type I would offer to do the mail or help someone else. I was determined to make a difference and treated my job as if it were the most important job in the company.

With my new job came another change in my life — moving out of my aunt's home. Aunt Edith was sad to see me go, but she understood that I needed to be out on my own. I had become the big sister to my three cousins and didn't want to lose contact with them, so I still went over once a week to have dinner and share with my aunt what was going on in my life. I moved into a one-bedroom apartment with a friend and a former co-worker from the bank, Shirley Ambrose. Shirley was also from Nova Scotia so we had a lot in common. Our small apartment became party central! Go-go boots and dancing on the tabletop at weekly parties in our apartment became the norm. We hung out at the Blue Spruce Hotel (yes, I was under age) and I loved dancing the night away. My world crumbled when the police asked me for I.D. one evening and I could no longer party with my older friends.

There were several things about living on my own that I still needed to learn. I didn't "do kitchen," and Shirley learned my lack of cooking skills rather quickly. The first night we were to make dinner together, I was put in charge of the potatoes. When Shirley came home I told her I had nearly burnt the apartment down, and showed her the blackened pot with the burnt potatoes. She suggested I had let the water burn off, and my reply was "Water? What water?" Mom had always been the cook at home and I had absolutely no desire to learn. I realized that cooking was not going to be my forte, and let Shirley be in charge of it from that point on.

In December of the same year I went home for Christmas, determined not to miss out on another family holiday.

Unfortunately, home was now a small, two-bedroom apartment in Annapolis Royal, half an hour away from Wilmot. The unthinkable had happened: my family had lost our beautiful home and Dad had lost his job. It was not the Christmas I had hoped for so desperately a few months ago. Mom had joined the Catholic Church in Annapolis Royal as soon as they moved and when she was not with my sisters she spent her time helping at the church. Often Mom could not afford to contribute to the Sunday collection plate. I believe by helping to clean the church she felt she was at least making a contribution.

The night I came home, a friend picked me up at the airport in Halifax and drove me to Annapolis Royal. Dad was so drunk I couldn't even wake him up to greet me; I left him passed out on the couch. Even though he was still in trouble financially, he continued to spend money like he had it. He had found a job as a mechanic at the local service station, but it barely paid the bills. That Christmas he wanted to get me a really nice gift since I was coming home all the way from North Bay. He criticized the beautiful blouse my mother had bought for me and decided to buy an expensive dresser set of a comb, brush, and mirror instead. He charged all the gifts, and less than a week later someone was at the door trying to collect the money. It was a very sad visit and a difficult Christmas. Lorraine and Connie were growing up and my heart ached for them both. They had been forced out of our home in Wilmot at a time in their lives when things should have been so much better.

When it was time for me to leave, I took Mom aside and begged her to keep me informed as much as possible. Mom said she would be fine, but did ask me to send change to Connie and Lorraine in my letters home. She didn't have the money to give them, but wanted them to have something of their own. It was so like Mom to be thinking of "her girls." I was terribly fearful about what would happen to all three of them.

I realized, more than ever before, how removed I was from everything that was going on with my family. Since we could only correspond through letters, I knew any bad news would be delayed by at least a week. It made me feel helpless and alone. Mom reassured me that she would be okay as I left to return to my life in North Bay. How was I to know that only months later her world would come crashing down around her?

Family Ties

$\mathcal{T}$he phone call came shortly after I had returned to North Bay. I was surprised to hear Lorraine's voice at the other end of the line as the operator asked if I would accept a collect call. My sister was fourteen years old, and I hardly had time to brace myself for what she was about to say.

"Dad's gone," she said. "He took all the money and gave Mom three dollars before he left. She is working in a restaurant. They don't pay her but they let her bring food home so she can feed us." Lorraine said the parish priest had been over to the apartment several times to talk with Mom about helping her find a paying job. I was shocked and frightened for all of them. Mom didn't know Lorraine was calling to tell me what had happened, but she said she would tell Mom we had talked. Lorraine knew I would want to hear immediately rather than reading it in a letter. Dad had told Mom he was going to look for work one day and would return soon, but he never came back. Before he left he withdrew the little bit of money they had in the bank and financed a new car. Mom didn't know about the car until she went to the bank to let them know Dad had left. She had to tell them not to come to her looking for repayment of his debts. Bill collectors had been coming to the apartment for days, and had already been telling Mom she wouldn't be able to keep anything in the apartment; they had even threatened to take my sisters' beds. Mom didn't have any money to continue renting the apartment, or to buy food for her and my sisters. I finished the conversation by promising Lorraine that I'd try to find a way to help them and that I'd write to Mom immediately.

Later that same day Mom called. She was sorry I had to hear such bad news, but was relieved that Lorraine had taken the initiative to make the call. She first told me not to worry and that her parish priest, Father Theriault, was going to help her find a job in Halifax. I think Mom's faith in the church was probably the only thing she had left at the time and it helped her focus on the future. All I could think about was that it was cowardly of my father to go off and leave Mom to deal with his debts. I felt terrible that I somehow couldn't have seen this coming after my visit home at Christmas. I told Mom I wanted to come home, that I was confident I could get a good job in Halifax. I wanted her to say she needed me to come home and help them, but her reply was reflective of her practical nature. She said while it would be great to have me there emotionally, they really needed me to help them financially; clearly I could make more money in North Bay than in Halifax. Mom went on to say that she felt more strongly now than ever that to come to Halifax as Perry Cole's daughter would ruin any chances of a career. Even if I could get a job, it would probably be the only one I would ever have since Dad's reputation had only gotten worse.

I was torn that my mother did not want me there, but comforted that she still needed me to help. At the time I had been promoted to a service representative at Bell, and was to travel to Sudbury on a six-week training course. During the course I would have an expense account and could send Mom most of my salary. Sometimes I would just put cash in an envelope and send it whenever I had some spare money. It was a very anxious time — I couldn't call them because there was no phone and I couldn't go home because I wanted to send them the money I would have spent getting there. Mom had agreed to call me collect twice a month, and we had some wonderful talks despite her situation. She would always ask about what was going on in North Bay and in my life. She would tell me funny stories about Lorraine and Connie and would convince me they were doing just fine. In fact, she was confident they were happier without my father being around. My mother could make the best of a bad situation and always found a way to give thanks and be positive. At the same time, these calls were difficult because I could tell from the strain in Mom's voice that she was having a hard time — she said little about how she was feeling personally.

Not long after Dad left, Mom knew he wasn't coming back, and made the decision to move to Halifax. Uncle Ralph and Aunt Eva helped Mom move her few belongings. Mom and Lorraine were going to stay with Lois until they found a place of their own. Connie stayed with the Whites in Wilmot for a few days, since Lois's one-bedroom apartment was busy with a new baby, her husband, and my mom and sister.

In Halifax, Father Theriault helped Mom find a job at the Halifax Infirmary — in the laundry department. Mom was fifty years old and had not worked outside the home since marrying Dad. Now this tiny woman was going to work in the sweltering hot laundry department helping to operate the large presses. When she started work that first Monday, all the Italian women who worked in the department wanted to know about Mom's husband. Mom found it funny that the main focus of conversation all day long was "their men." Eventually Mom began to form friendships with these women and they were very supportive of her over the years.

As soon as Mom had a job, she began to look for a place for the three of them to live. The only thing they could afford initially was one room in a small rundown apartment building, where they had to share a fridge and a washroom with other families. Mom made the best of it with her girls — her goal was to keep them together as a family, raise them properly, and be the very best mother she could be. Since Mom couldn't give the girls spending money, I would continue to send them weekly letters with change attached to them. Connie and Lorraine would have to pull the change off carefully if they wanted to read the letter. One day Mom wrote and asked me to stop sending Connie the "change" letters. Apparently she was not reading the letter, but just ripping off the change. When Mom told me this I marvelled at her strength — she was not in a position to say no to the money, yet she did not want my sisters to develop bad habits.

While Mom was undergoing so much turmoil in Halifax, I found myself caught up in a whirlwind of excitement in North Bay. I had fallen in love with Graydon Scott. Graydon was in the air force and was stationed in North Bay. It was shocking for me to experience the trauma at home on the one hand, and be enjoying my own life on the other. I broke a cardinal girlfriend's rule by dating Graydon: I went out with someone my roommate had already dated, although Shirley really didn't care. Graydon was actually engaged to a girl in Europe at the time, so I was determined to change his mind. It was love at first sight for me and Graydon was my everything. I loved everything about him . . . except that he was already engaged. He finally broke off the relationship with his fiancée, we became intimate, and as a good Catholic girl the next thing I had to do was to marry. We were engaged in the fall of 1966 and I went to his home in Belleville that Christmas to meet his family. I loved all of them, especially his sister Gaye, who would become a friend for life. We set the date for our wedding: August 5, 1967. I was hopelessly in love with Graydon and just wanted to get married as soon as possible. I knew my mom and my sisters would not be able to attend because of their financial situation, and I couldn't afford to bring them to the wedding, so I settled on the next best thing. We would go to Halifax on our honeymoon. Then I could tell Mom and my sisters all about the wedding in person and spend some time visiting.

We got married on the air force base and Shirley Ambrose was my maid of honour. It was a day of mixed emotions — I had never been so in love and was thrilled to be Graydon's wife. But when a telegram from Mom was read during the reception, I could not stop crying. I missed my family. Graydon understood and told me he was as anxious as I was to go to Halifax. He was always very accepting of the fact that I was helping my mom financially. He never questioned my decision, and knew how close my relationship was with my family.

We stopped at Expo '67 in Montreal on the way, and had a wonderful time, but I couldn't wait to continue driving to Nova Scotia. I was so anxious to get home that the full reality of my mother's situation didn't hit me in the face until I saw where they were living. Mom was still in the one-room apartment with Connie and Lorraine. Graydon and I were staying in a hotel not far from the apartment and the first morning we awoke to a knock on the door very early. "Tell me that is not your sisters already," Graydon said, but I knew my two very happy sisters were on the other side of the door. Even more exhilarating for Connie was the treat that Mom had bought for my homecoming. "We have peaches to go with supper tonight!" she shouted. I was so happy to see them but it was also very sad for me. I could afford all the peaches I wanted and to see my sister so excited about something that I took for granted really upset me. It broke my heart to see Mom and all her possessions in that one shabby room.

I had mailed Mom pictures of my wedding while we were on our way to Halifax. We went through the entire wedding day with her and my sisters. From picture to picture I tried to recreate the whole experience for them. I know it was difficult for Mom to see the pictures, as I imagine it would have been for any mother who didn't attend her daughter's wedding. It took me a very long time to forgive myself for not having her at my wedding.

That particular visit home was a turning point for me in terms of the relationship I had with my mother. As with many women who get married, the focus in my life became my marriage and it shifted away from my mother and sisters. I didn't go home for Christmas every year or visit every summer after that. I continued to help Mom financially as much as I could.

She kept working at the Halifax Infirmary, and eventually she was able to save enough money to move out of the one-room apartment and into a very nice place.

When I met Graydon I was enjoying my new promotion to a residential service representative at Bell. After the six-week training course I took in Sudbury, I arrived back in North Bay determined to continue moving up the Bell ladder. I really loved the job. I loved communicating with people, listening to them, and helping them. When I started the position my talkative nature was a bit of a problem. For the first few months as a service representative, managers monitor your calls to make sure you are giving out the right information and treating customers properly. Whenever I felt I wanted to say something that was outside of the training rules, I always checked to see if the managers were listening in on the calls. One day I had a rather unpleasant customer on the phone who wanted to have an extension telephone installed. She was very upset that it would take three days before the extension could be installed in her house and was griping about the service charge. During that particular week, the service charge was changing from six dollars on the Thursday to nine dollars on the Friday. I had really had enough of this woman's complaining and when she asked me what the service charge would be, I replied: "Actually, I have good news and bad news. The good news is, if we come before Thursday it will only cost you six dollars. The bad news is, we can't come until Friday."

As soon as I made the remark I saw out of the corner of my eye one of the managers coming out of the monitoring room. She motioned for me to finish the conversation and then flipped the switch so I would not receive any more calls. She herded me into her office.

"Carol Ann, what are you doing? That was totally unprofessional of you. You can't just say anything you want."

"But I made her laugh," I protested. My manager then mentioned that magic word — career — and I became more serious. She reminded me that if I wanted a career with Bell I had to show a serious side. It could not be fun all the time and, so far, I seemed mainly interested in making people laugh. I resolved on the spot to be less of a smart aleck.

Shortly after completing my residential service rep's course my managers decided that I should take the business service rep's course. I would now be able to take calls from the business community in North Bay in addition to my other responsibilities. Carolyn Passmore had moved on to be a training instructor and we would work together, one on one. It became a game for me to see how much I could learn each day; Carolyn was an excellent teacher. She pushed me and understood that I always wanted her to give me more and more to do. We completed the course in record time and I felt a great sense of achievement. My job as services representative allowed me to make more than the $56.50 a week I had started with. Every three months brought a raise in pay and I felt I had proven the rumour to be true — you *can* make more money in Ontario. I was now earning over ninety dollars per week, which was a regular fortune to me. The regular salary increases allowed me to see the potential for making some serious money if I continued to be promoted. The money also allowed me to help my mother and sisters in different ways.

Even though I didn't go home to Halifax on a regular basis, I was able to see my sisters every summer when they would visit us in North Bay. Their visits provided a nice break for Mom, especially when they were all living in one room. I loved spending time with Connie and Lorraine and it was also a chance to see how their personalities were developing. I wish I could say my marriage was strong at that time, but both Connie and Lorraine could see that ours was not a happy home. It bothered me that after what they had been through with Dad they were now catching a glimpse of my unhappy marriage.

Soon after we were married, I realized that Graydon and I were on an entirely different page when it came to work. A job was a job for Graydon, while I wanted a career. The lifestyle I wanted was very different from the one we had. Most of the people we hung out with were military couples. Air force wives were just that — wives of the important men in the air force. They didn't even use their first name, but went by their husband's name. It was Mrs. John Doe, not even Jane Doe, and I could not understand why any woman would do that. Many of these women would talk exclusively about their husband's needs and wants and ignore their own feelings. Only a few of them worked outside of the home and it was obvious I didn't fit in with them at all — nor did I try to. I remember one couple coming over for dinner (we must have ordered in). The husband was in the service with Graydon and his wife stayed home and kept the house, which was the way he wanted it. Graydon said, "Not Carol Ann — she thinks the business world needs her. She thinks she *has* to work, and is going to make more money than me one day." I was the only person in the room who didn't find Graydon's comment funny. I felt totally suffocated by the air force mentality at that time. My social life seemed to consist of watching Graydon participate in sports or watching a movie at the base with the other wives. I began to question my goals and dreams of having a career, thinking that maybe my priorities were all wrong and I should start acting like the other wives. I decided to shift my focus to my marriage and the possibility of motherhood.

We decided to have a child after we had been married for two years. When I think back now, the way that we made our decision to have a child was ridiculous. We were driving to Florida and decided that if we could afford to go on this vacation, then we could afford to have a child. In a moment of carefree abandon I threw my birth control pills out the car window — on April 1. I became pregnant on that trip and Jamie was born exactly nine months later on January 1, 1969. My nickname for Jamie was "the boy." An interesting coincidence was that my best friend Donna gave birth to her son two weeks after Jamie was born. Donna and I still kept in touch and I always found her to be a very levelling influence. She married her high school sweetheart and decided to be a stay-at-home mother after Scott and Tasha were born. Our regular letters helped us both through our new motherhood jitters.

When I was pregnant I made the decision to quit my job at Bell. At that time a maternity leave wasn't offered, but you could take a leave of absence. I decided I would just quit, since I was going to focus all my energy on being Mother and Wife of the Year. Once I perfected that, I might think about working again. At the time, I had no idea how much I would miss working.

Soon after Jamie was born, I realized I had to get out of the house and do some type of work; just a couple of hours a day might be enough to make me feel more connected with people. I decided to become an Avon lady. I strapped Jamie to my chest in a contraption that I made out of flannelette sheets — who knew I could have made a fortune years later if I had patented that baby holder. Selling Avon was a job; it got me out of the house and gave me some spending money (Mom and my sisters had every single product Avon sold). But I knew Avon wasn't really the calling I was looking for, and it would never substitute for a career. This realization hit me one day when I rang the doorbell and a man whom I had once dated opened the door. He was home visiting his mother and was surprised to see me. The first thing he said was, "This is what became of you, you're an Avon lady?"

As soon as the words were out of his mouth and he saw the look on my face, he immediately tried to backtrack and said, "Not that there's anything wrong with what you're doing, but I didn't think you would end up as an Avon lady." At that moment I realized that the person I wanted to be had *not* disappeared from my life. I immediately went home and waited for Graydon to come home from work. As soon as he walked through the door I told him that I had decided to return to work. I had been selling Avon for four months and told him I just didn't find being a wife and mother fulfilling enough. Graydon agreed I should go back to work, especially if I wasn't happy.

Going back to my job at Bell was not as easy as I had hoped. There was a problem: some of the people I had once worked with did not want me back. When I asked Martin Kennelly for a job he arranged to meet me outside of the office so we could talk. When I arrived for the meeting I was surprised to see Carolyn Passmore there as well. They both wanted to be brutally honest with me and let me know that since I had quit, a lot of the service representatives thought I shouldn't get my old job back. Apparently some saw me as a bit of a troublemaker, gossiping when I should have been working and spending too much time trying to make people laugh. Even more daunting for some of these women was the prospect that I might have a shot at a management position. They felt that would be unfair since I had quit. It was so hard for me to hear the criticisms. I was unhappy in my marriage, I had very few friends, and now I was being reminded (and rightly so) that I may not have been the best employee. I vowed to learn from this experience and move forward. I wanted to go back and prove myself after receiving this feedback, and eventually I did return to Bell. Kathy and Bill Service were our best friends outside of Graydon's air force friends and Kathy worked with me at Bell. She found a way to support me when I returned to work and slowly I became more confident around the women I knew I had disappointed.

Two years after Jamie was conceived, April 1, 1970, I returned to work, and two months later was promoted to the position of acting manager. As I became enmeshed in my work life again, I realized that my marriage was not going to work. When I made the decision to go back to work I knew it might contribute to the break-up of my marriage, but I also knew that my career would allow me to strike out on my own if necessary. Graydon and I were not acknowledging we were unhappy together; instead we would just avoid doing things together, and the focus became "the boy." We could sit in a room with Jamie and never look at each other, speaking through our son if anything needed to be said. It was a very sad and lonely time. Two people can often be lonelier than one; I was learning this the hard way.

I remember vividly the day I finally admitted not only to myself, but to someone else that my marriage was over. Mr. Kennelly came over to my desk one Friday afternoon and said, "I see the North Bay Tiger Cats are out of town this weekend. Would you like to leave work early today to go with your husband?" Graydon was a member of the team and a minor celebrity in town, and this was such a touching gesture on Mr. Kennelly's part. I started to cry and said, "I'm leaving Graydon." He took me into his office, closed the door, and asked me if I had told anyone in the office. I shook my head tearfully. I felt that I just couldn't tell them, given the fact that all the people in my office had been to my wedding.

"We are your family here and you should tell them before they hear about it from someone else," he told me gently.

I will be forever thankful to Mr. Kennelly for giving me a great deal of guidance during that period. He took me to see a lawyer in our building, so I would know what legal actions to take. He was also concerned about my emotional state and made me schedule an appointment with my doctor right away. Next, he took me to see my parish priest since I was troubled by the fact that a divorce would prevent me from receiving communion in the Catholic Church. The priest at my church confirmed that I could not leave my husband. Instead of taking that as a final answer, Mr. Kennelly drove me to another priest just outside of North Bay. In those days I guess you would have called him a bit of a hippie priest (his hair was almost covering his ears!). He gave me some advice that was very profound. He did agree that the Catholic Church says if you leave your husband, you might go to hell.

"But the way I see it, if you stay with him you are living in hell now — so pay now or pay later," he said with a smile. I loved his rationale.

Graydon and I had discussed our marriage all we cared to, and had mutually agreed that it was over, and it was time to get on with our separate lives. When it came time to discuss moving arrangements, we decided that because I would take care of Jamie, it would be important for Jamie to stay at the house. So Graydon prepared to move out.

Instead of thinking about the magnitude of my problems, I focussed on breaking free of the unhappy feelings I had had for so long. After I told Mr. Kennelly and made the decision to go ahead with a divorce, I wrote my mother telling her that Graydon and I were splitting up. It was a very long letter. When Connie picked up the mail a week later she rushed over to the infirmary where Mom was working, thinking my letter contained lots of new pictures. Mom realized what the letter was about, and she was very upset. That night she called me to talk. Mom wanted to reassure me that everything would be okay, and that she had the confidence I could carry on. We cried together on the phone as she gave me lots of advice. I knew that Mom worried about not being there to support me emotionally, but even talking on the phone with her lifted my spirits. If my mom could carry on with what she was doing, raising Connie and Lorraine while working at a physically exhausting job, I had nothing to be worried about. I was still young at twenty-five, had a good job, and was financially able to care for my son.

At the time it was not common to see many working single mothers at Bell. Most employees were either married or still single and dating. Single was not "in" if you had a child. For the longest time, my family and friends would think they were comforting me by saying, "Don't worry, he'll come back." They would even spell the word F-A-T-H-E-R rather than say it in front of my son, thinking Jamie would be upset. I finally had to put a stop to this nonsense by replying, "Jamie has a father, but we are not together," or "Graydon didn't die, we just got divorced." Instead of being depressed about getting a divorce,

I felt invigorated. The day Graydon moved out of the house, I rearranged the furniture, trying to remove his presence from "my" space. Jamie helped by moving bricks from one side of the living room to the other so we could rebuild our bookcase. He felt important with this job and with much grunting and groaning he moved over 100 bricks — one at a time — all by himself. Everything of Graydon's was either packed away or thrown out; not out of malice, but in an attempt to make a clean start.

I knew I could do this. I would find a way to balance both my ambitions for a career with caring for Jamie. Somehow I would have my "big job at the Bell" and win a Mother of the Year award too! It would be the beginning of Jamie and I growing up together.

"The Boy"

$\mathcal{I}$ knew when Jamie was born that babies did not come with a manual, but I also knew I was not going to be a mother in the traditional sense. In all my years I had never done things by the book, and I was proud to think that the conventions of motherhood might also be different for me.

Jamie's birth was very difficult for me physically, and I was in isolation for a few days. While most mothers are able to hold their baby right away, I had to wait days until he was brought to me. He was very long, skinny, and bruised from the birth. I didn't expect the response I had the first time I held him. Here was a being who really needed me — and at that stage in my life I think I needed him just as much. I had left my family at home in circumstances I couldn't control, my marriage was not what I expected, and my career path was still shaky. But Jamie's birth really grounded me in realizing I now had a focus as a mother.

My need for a "motherhood manual" became evident the first time I took Jamie out. He was three weeks old and I was eager to show him off, just "the boy" and me. Exercise classes were held at a local school and we were the first to arrive. I carefully arranged him on the floor of the gym with my winter coat covering all but his eyes and nose. My concentration then moved to my friends arriving one by one saying, "Look at you — you've got your flat stomach back already!" (I think I went to show off my figure as much as my new son.) The exercise class began and finished. Finally someone said, "Carol Ann, I thought you would have brought your son to show him off." I had forgotten all about him! I panicked as I looked over to the corner where I had left him. On top of my coat — which was on top of him — were the heavy winter coats belonging to everyone who had come to the class. I ran over, dug him out from under the pile, and held him high in the air shouting "presenting James Brian Scott — 'the boy.'" One of the air force wives felt the need to remind me that life was no longer about me and my flat stomach. I must now put my son's needs before my own. Lesson learned.

Jamie brought a new kind of euphoria to my life. He was a happy child and I loved to show him off. We even had a "trick" we performed together. Jamie really hated eating carrots. His entire little body would shiver if he ate even one spoonful. When Graydon and I had company I would show them Jamie's trick. I would give him a spoonful of applesauce (to fool him) and then a spoonful of carrots. He would shiver, and everyone thought it was funny, including Jamie.

Jamie started going to nursery school shortly after I returned to work. The daycare centre was always filled with children and he loved playing there every day. Many of the mothers who worked at Bell dropped their kids off each morning as I did. After I separated from Graydon, I felt I was constantly scrutinized for how long Jamie spent there. He was the first child to be dropped off in the morning and usually the last one to be picked up at the end of the day, waiting for me with his nose pressed against the window. The daycare staff would always make comments like, "*Finally*, here she comes." I quickly realized how different life would be. I knew it was going to be a challenge trying to balance my career and being a single mother. By that time I had been promoted to a first-level manager at Bell, and was once again considering getting back on the career path full time. We didn't own a car, so we would have a long walk home from the daycare centre every day. Jamie was always happy to see me and eager to begin our walk home. He would run into the fields chasing birds, making the long walk even longer. He could almost catch up to a bird, but then he would say something to me and the bird would fly away. Undaunted, he would walk in the direction the bird had flown rather than back to me.

On our way home we would stop at a convenience store for milk or bread. Jamie would always ask me for a treat. We didn't have any money to spare, so I developed a game to keep Jamie occupied. I told him that we would take turns being the "treat" — one day he could be the treat and the next day I would be the treat. Each day before we entered the store he would ask, "Who's the treat today?" One day when I was especially tired and cranky with him, Jamie quickly told me it was my turn to be the treat. I turned to him and said sarcastically, "Yeah, I'm a *real* treat today." Jamie stood talking to a few people from the neighbourhood while I bought the milk. As I approached them I heard my neighbour say, "Here comes your mother." Without missing a beat, the first thing that popped out of Jamie's mouth was, "Yeah, she's a *real* treat today."

Jamie and I talked about everything. He was living in an adult world with me and I chose to speak with him as I would any other adult. As we walked home together each day we would talk about my job and his day with the kids. He could ask a very innocent question about my day and I could see how trivial my problems were through the eyes of a child. I was often amazed and very proud of the adult-like way he could carry a conversation.

On my twenty-fifth birthday I took the day off work and kept Jamie home from nursery school. I wanted to talk with him about our future. It had been a roller coaster two years since his birth. A year earlier, in 1970, when the Apollo 13 mission was called a "successful failure," I began to think of my marriage that way — with Jamie being the success. I talked with him about us being not alone, but *together* as we moved forward with our lives. I explained that it would be tough and lonely and that I really didn't even know how we would get through it. I cried while he tried to work his magic into the conversation. Jamie loved to use two different phrases at that stage of his young life and he often confused them. Instead of saying, "I don't mind," or "It doesn't matter," he would mix them up and say, "I don't matter," or "It doesn't mind." That particular day I explained that we would not be living with his dad, we wouldn't have a car, we would have to walk to the laundromat each week, and Mommy would have to work very hard to make more money. I was totally negative in that moment, seeing all the things we *wouldn't* have as a result of the divorce. Jamie looked at me, saw my tears, and quietly said, "Don't cry

Mommy, it doesn't mind." And, you know, it really didn't mind.

I was gaining my confidence back at work day by day, and the promotion to first-level manager was just the beginning. As a manager I knew I liked running the show: helping people and taking responsibility for what went well and what didn't during the day. I also realized there was not much further for me to go in the small North Bay office. I think both Mr. Kennelly and Carolyn Passmore knew I wanted more from my career, too. One day Mr. Kennelly called me in to his office and asked, "Are you mobile?" At first I thought he was asking if I lived in a mobile home! He explained that if I would be willing to move to another city he could find opportunities for me to advance my career elsewhere. He felt I was ready for more responsibility than his office could offer me and he was encouraging me to think beyond my life in North Bay. This was so exciting to hear. I knew I could do so much more.

I was preparing to go to British Columbia to visit my sister Lois, her husband, and two daughters. I was dating a man named Gordon McGuinty, and this would be our first vacation together. As soon as we arrived, Lois told me they were moving to Kingston — only a few hours from North Bay. I was so excited, since it would be the first time in my adult life I would have a family member close by. It was not as hard to say good-bye to Lois when my vacation ended, because I knew I would be seeing her more often. What I didn't realize was that after our pre-vacation conversation, Mr. Kennelly had submitted my name for a job opening in Kingston. As soon as I returned to work, I told him about Lois moving to Kingston. A week later, I was shocked when he called me into his office and asked if I was interested in being even closer to my sister. He then told me I was being transferred to Kingston as a second-level manager. I would be in charge of the COB — the combined order bureau — and all of the managers and typists would report to me. It would be an entirely female team.

"Congratulations, kid, you are on your way. They want you there in two weeks," he said with a twinkle in his eye. I could tell he was proud of me when he made the announcement to the rest of the staff in the office. Everyone was very supportive, especially Carolyn, who had been such a big help during my "ups-and-downs" in the office.

I knew I was ready for this new job and all its challenges, but the relocation terrified me. It was hard to put my feelings into words as my job promotion was announced. In the year since my separation from Graydon, I had begun to have a more positive sense of who I was and what I wanted to accomplish. I had become confident that I could raise Jamie properly, have a successful career, and a social life. I was proud of who I was becoming. At the same time, it was hard to imagine leaving the security of North Bay, a town where so much had occurred in the nine years I had lived there. And this would be my first move as a single parent. With so many responsibilities, I wondered how I would manage. Two weeks did not give me much time — my list of things to do (I make daily lists) would be a long one.

That evening Jamie and I set out on our Friday night "date." This had become a regular weekly event for us. We went to the Ponderosa restaurant where Jamie always ordered his meal by number — his favourite was a number four. I wanted to share my good news, and feeling an "upscale restaurant" was in order, we dressed up and set out to celebrate. The waitress fell in love with Jamie and read the entire menu to him. Thinking he had understood she asked, "What would you like, my dear?" Very confidently Jamie replied, "Do you gots a number four?" As we enjoyed our dinner, I told him Mommy had been promoted and we would be moving to Kingston in two weeks. To make it more exciting for him, I told him we would try to have him promoted as well — from nursery school to school! He was almost five years old and I felt he needed to be with older children because he had been in nursery school for so long. I knew accomplishing this would be a struggle because the "rule" said a child must turn five by December 31. Jamie was a New Year's baby, so technically he was one day too late to start school that September.

I had to explain my career goals and the move to Gordon as well. He was very supportive, but wondered if a move to Kingston was necessary. Our relationship was fairly new and the distance between cities was a concern to both of us. We vowed to make it all work out and he promised to make the drive to Kingston every weekend.

I took a week off work and Jamie and I went to Kingston to begin our new life. I turned it into an adventure for him: we stayed in a motel and each day we would get on our bikes and cycle around. I knew I had to find a school, a babysitter, and an apartment all within a couple of days. The first day in Kingston we rode around different neighbourhoods looking for the right school. I wanted Jamie to go to a Catholic school. In retrospect the way I approached that first move may have been a bit backwards; initially I should have looked for an apartment. But I was determined to get Jamie into a good school and thought that was the most important thing to find first. I knew it might be difficult, but I didn't realize just *how* hard it was going to be. Because of his birthday, the Catholic school board wouldn't enrol him. They did not want to bend the rules. I did.

It was the first battle that I fought in Kingston as a single mother. I played my cards all wrong the first time I spoke with the school board, telling them I was a single mother and would be travelling with this new job at Bell and really needed Jamie to be in school. I'm sure it sounded like I was begging, but I wanted Jamie to have interaction with other kids his age; he was simply too old for daycare. The Catholic school board was not thrilled to hear that I was a divorced, single mother and all they wanted to talk about was my husband. I kept reminding them Graydon was not part of this team. It was Jamie and I. At one point the teacher turned to me and said sarcastically, "So you're divorced — but you *are* Catholic, correct?" Jamie was sitting on her lap, bouncing on her knee. He looked up at her and said, "We're Catholic, but we don't go to church." I was sure that would be the end of the discussion. However, I think the teacher now saw it as the school's duty to help him and hopefully direct both of us back to church. He could start school in September.

With Jamie enrolled in school we were now ready to look for an apartment and a babysitter. We found the babysitter by cycling around the neighbourhood and talking with young mothers we saw outside. One of them was Viola, who was sitting on her steps with her young boys. I stopped to ask her if she knew anyone who babysat, as I was new to the area. Jamie had gotten off his bike and was already talking with her boys. It was obvious they were getting along well. Jamie was always a magnet for kids and adults alike. He loved to talk — much like his mother — and could always make friends easily. Viola offered to look after Jamie after school during the week. It was a relief to find someone who so obviously loved children. Equally as important, her boys really liked having Jamie around.

They almost became a second family to Jamie when I travelled on business. For any single mother, finding the right babysitter is the most important task of all. I was very fortunate.

With two of our tasks completed, we now turned our attention to finding an apartment. My goal was to find an apartment building with a washer and dryer. Ultimately I wanted to *own* a washer and dryer, but that was still in our future. Just being able to do laundry without leaving the building would be a bonus. In North Bay I was making $10,000 and the promotion moved me up to $13,000 a year. An increase that gave me a salary of more than $1,000 per month seemed huge and, for a moment, I felt rich. However, I quickly learned that rent was going to be more than I expected in Kingston, and we would only be able to afford a basement apartment. We found one in a beautiful building on Killendale Avenue, close to Jamie's school. I was thrilled that a washer and dryer were included — even if I didn't own them myself. On top of the higher rent, I now found myself with additional babysitting costs. Although Lois was in Kingston, she lived on the air base with her family — a great distance from our apartment and Jamie's school. I was expected to represent Bell on many occasions in the community and did not like to rely on Viola for evening babysitting. Lois was unable to look after Jamie during the week and I had to depend on babysitters often.

My leap into the second level of management at Bell was into quite a different environment than my earlier job in North Bay. As a female manager in the 1970s, even at that junior level, I felt I had to work harder than my male counterparts. Just to ensure that I understood my position in terms of ranking with my male peers, many colleagues told me that women would not be promoted beyond this level. Managing the typing pool might be as good as it would get. My predecessor had been a woman as well, but she had left on maternity leave and the reaction of the men was that Bell would not make that "mistake" again. In fact, one of the managers lost a case of beer in a bet that they would not bring another female manager into the position. I learned about the bet after I arrived and offered to buy Mark a beer since he had lost out on a whole case. Laughing with them was sometimes the best way to work with the male mentality of the era.

With this new job came another level of expectation: extracurricular activities, which required sitting on different boards and representing Bell on numerous committees. Women often had to do more to be considered equal with the men and Kingston was the first lesson in that arena for me. I knew it, and I was happy to play the game to prove I deserved to be there. My boss at the time was very helpful in pointing out the types of committees I should be sitting on. As a female manager I knew I had to take it one step further. I had to do more than he suggested. At any one given time I worked with at least four groups — the Business and Professional Women's Club in Kingston, the local Council for Women, the Board of Trade, and the Junior Chamber of Commerce. I was also involved in Career Day for women at Queen's University and tried to mentor women considering a career in business. I wanted everyone to share my commitment to a career. In fact, I wanted everyone to work at Bell! I loved working with all these groups. Additionally, it gave me a chance to connect with other women in the community.

I can admit now, these numerous commitments did wear me out at times. It was easier for my male co-workers to fulfil all of these duties since most of their wives were home to look after their families and households. It was obvious there were different standards for men and women. I had to bite my tongue one Monday morning when my boss suggested a male peer of mine should have stayed home to rest. Apparently his wife had been ill and he had spent the weekend looking after the house, the family, and completing all the chores by himself. I wanted to jump up and yell, "Hello! Let me tell you about *my* weekend!" But to do so would have been a professional disaster. Double standards clearly existed, but it was not for me to point them out.

Weekdays at our home were very busy and evenings even more so. I would pick Jamie up at Viola's after work and hurry home to feed him and spend some time together before the evening babysitter arrived. Most of my meetings were from eight until nine or ten at night, so by the time I got home Jamie would be fast asleep. I felt guilty about seeing Jamie very little from Monday through Thursday. There were times where I just paused and asked myself, "What on earth am I doing and how much longer am I going to do this?" Although I was extremely focused on my career, I did worry about what impact this lifestyle was having on Jamie. The mind of a child never ceases to amaze me though, and Jamie took everything in stride.

When I had to make overnight business trips to Toronto during the week, Jamie would stay at Viola's house. Viola and her husband always treated Jamie as if he were a member of their own family. They loved having him around and I was grateful for the loving relationship he had with them. Jamie always looked upon these sleepovers as a treat, the chance to hang out with their boys. He would pack his pyjamas and clothes in a paper bag and I would drop him off at Viola's in the morning before school.

One morning as we were walking to the car Jamie struck up a conversation with a neighbour. "Guess what I have in this bag?" he asked. "My pyjamas, because my mother won't come home tonight," he said, shrieking with laughter.

Everyone in my neighbourhood knew I was a single mother, but they sometimes wrongly assumed that I was off gallivanting with a man. They would ask if I had a good night planned and it never crossed their minds to ask me otherwise. In the 1970s, people rarely assumed it was career-related, even though I would stress my overnight trips were business meetings in Toronto. I even lost one babysitter for Jamie because of my supposed "meetings." My sitter's husband felt there was no way a woman would be as busy as I said I was at work, and that it would be wrong for them to continue looking after my son. A week later my name was mentioned in the local paper and her husband had a change of heart. She called me back to apologize for their mistake, but I never let her babysit Jamie again.

When I was away on weekends, Jamie would stay with Lois and her family. She would cook him wonderful meals with desserts of chocolate-sauce-on-anything, take him on excursions, and include him as part of her family. He got to know his cousins, Natalie and Dawn Marie. It was wonderful to be close to my sister again and having her in Kingston was a godsend for me.

Gordon made the trip to visit us most weekends and during the winters in Kingston he introduced us to skiing. Gordon was an elite in the ski world and Jamie developed a passion for the sport. When Gordon wasn't with us, my life in Kingston — aside from Jamie — was all about work. Whether it was going to meetings, talking at schools, or putting in extra hours on the weekend, I knew I wanted that next promotion. I felt

I was at the bottom of the ladder and wanted to start climbing. It was not until I moved to Kingston that I realized the potential job opportunities that existed in Ottawa and Toronto. The thought of moving to Toronto terrified me, but I felt Ottawa might be a great place to live. I talked with my boss often and expressed my desire to move. I felt ready for a promotion and knew it would not happen in Kingston. At the end of my second year in Kingston, I was transferred to Ottawa in a lateral job — same level, more money.

Jamie and I had our Friday evening date and I explained we were moving to Ottawa. This time we had saved a bit of money and I hoped we would be buying our first home — a condo would suit our lifestyle perfectly. I explained to Jamie that if we did make a purchase he should invest some of his money. He was not keen to part with half of his life savings — he had $200 in the bank. But in the end he agreed to try it. He would invest some of his money in the initial down payment, and with every move we'd make thereafter, he'd double his original investment. It was a great way to teach him about investing his money.

Graydon had remarried and Jamie now had three stepbrothers (although he always thought of them as brothers). Graydon's wife, Christine, was wonderful with Jamie and I marvelled at how she treated him as "one of the boys" so easily. She would buy new clothes for him when she shopped for her sons and always made him feel part of her life. That summer, Christine bought Jamie new jeans just before he left and explained that his mom would have to hem them. He told her that he would take them to his tailor. He wasn't bragging, he just knew that if we needed something hemmed, it went to the tailor, *not* Mom.

Growing up, Jamie always spent his entire summer vacations with Graydon, Christine, Paul, Michael, and Sean. We later admitted to each other that these summers provided a welcome change for both of us. The time apart was good for our relationship and helped us appreciate each other more when he would come home to start school each September. It also helped his relationship with his dad continue to grow over the years.

We purchased our first condo — both Jamie and I. We had a wonderful home *and* our very own washer and dryer. Jamie adapted quickly to the move, loving the fact that we lived in a condo with a pool. We stood on our balcony with great excitement waiting for the moving van to drive down Baseline Road. Jamie went downstairs immediately to meet the movers, and asked if they could find his bike. I had been so focused on unpacking that it was several hours later when I asked the movers if Jamie was in their way. One of the movers said, "No, Jamie asked us to give you the message that he has gone to school." I had enrolled him in school already, and had driven him by the building to show him where he would be going in September. I worried about him as I continued to unpack boxes and when he came home at lunchtime I said, "Jamie, where have you been?" He quietly replied, "Did you not get my message? I went to school. You showed me where it was, remember?" He was going to be away all summer and had been keen to see what his new school looked like. Jamie was taking charge of his life at such a young age, learning to take on his own responsibilities and acting like an adult.

In Ottawa I once again threw myself into the job. Jamie still had to spend a lot of time at the babysitter's after school, but I would occasionally bring him into the office after work and on the weekends. There were always some co-workers in the office and they all loved talking with Jamie. He would often ask me on Friday evening if "we" were working on the weekend — meaning, could he go to the office with me. With the move to Ottawa, Jamie began to understand a little bit more what it was like to have a mother who worked. One day he came home from school upset and said, "None of my friends or teachers ever asks me what you do. They all want to know what my father does." It was a line that he was to hear over and over again growing up. Jamie felt his mom was special because she had what she had been calling for years her "big job at the Bell." It would be a few more years before he realized that not all moms carried a briefcase, had meetings in other cities, and worked weekends. In one of the few instances I was ill, Jamie came home for lunch instead of going to the sitter's house. It was such a novelty to him to have his mother home during the day. He asked me very seriously, "Mom, what grade will I be in when you are home every day?" Ah, the guilt that comes with motherhood.

One of the things that never changed during Jamie's years of growing up was my lack of interest in cooking meals for us at home. Since my blackened potato incident I had never cooked. We would order take-out or I would pick up a simple meal at the market on the way home. Many nights I would pick Jamie up from the sitter's after school, stop at a restaurant to eat, and then we would go back to the office for a few hours. These were the days before pre-made meals, and even those probably would have been too much for me to handle. We rarely sat at our dining room table and a big meal meant we went to a nice restaurant. Jamie only protested once about our arrangement, when he was still very young. He had been visiting his dad over the holidays and when he came back to Ottawa I told him I wanted to throw a special party for his birthday. I suggested he could invite a bunch of his friends and we would all go to a restaurant. He looked at me with a pained expression and said, "Can we stay home for once?"

Jamie definitely grew up on pizza and I finally had to admit that I would never win the Mother of the Year award for that aspect of his life. When he was sixteen years old and we were living in Toronto, we were walking down Yonge Street when we passed a pizza delivery guy. Mr. Pizza turned around, walked up to us, and tapped Jamie on the chest saying, "Hey I know you, your address is 71 Charles Street," and continued on his way. Not something a mother can brag about, although we still laugh when we tell the story today.

We were growing up together as I had predicted. Jamie and I were developing a wonderful and unique relationship; while his upbringing was very different from that of his friends, I know he enjoyed every minute of it. Our moves to Kingston and Ottawa would be two of many more as I climbed that corporate ladder — with Jamie by my side every step of the way. As I celebrated my thirtieth birthday I contemplated my next promotion and my ultimate goal — to be a vice president before my fortieth birthday.

10 South

On November 1, 1976, Jamie and I were celebrating my latest promotion. Not only had I been promoted, but the job was still in Ottawa so we did not face another move — yet. Jamie was seven years old and still able to describe my job using his own language. He listened as I talked about my new position and my team of male peers, and asked what level this job would be. I proudly explained I would now be a third-level manager. His reply once again put things in perspective: "So, now we're both in Grade Three!"

Mom and my younger sisters came to celebrate Christmas with us and it was so special to have our family together in my new home. Lois and her family joined us from Kingston. I was proud of what Mom had accomplished on her own. She had entered the work force at fifty and now could talk about retiring with a pension when she turned sixty-five. She had come so far! Mom joked that at the pace I was keeping I wouldn't last until I turned sixty-five. She said I should start thinking of retiring early. I promised to think about it.

At the office I was settling into my new job, but soon discovered the drawbacks of being a female in a higher position of management. During a regular monthly meeting, we were discussing what job aids were required to improve productivity in the work force. The talk turned to one of my peers who had been transferred from an Installation and Repair District to the Business Office, which meant he would now be supervising a female work force rather than a male-dominated one. One of my peers passed a note around the room to the other men. They were all snickering and enjoying the joke immensely. While they made no move to hide what was going on, they certainly did not feel the need to share it with the only female in the room. I tried to ignore what was going on, but when we had a washroom break, I took the note out of the garbage before they returned. The note was written to my peer who would be supervising the female-dominated business office. It read, "The only job aid you're going to need is a large jar of Vaseline. Enjoy your new job." I was shocked that every one of those men had found it so funny and took such pleasure in laughing in front of me. For one instant, I thought, "I can do this job, but I'm not sure I want to work with these men." As they all filed back into the room, my shock turned to anger and I briefly considered confronting them. Instead I quietly folded the note, tucked it away, and continued the meeting. I felt completely powerless because I knew that if I said something to my boss it was still going to be me versus them. Since I was new to third-level management, I knew my boss would probably tell me to get a thicker skin, that it was only a joke. I would appear weak in their eyes. I carried that note around for many months before I threw it away. It was symbolic of just how condescending men could be to women climbing the corporate ladder.

I have always been the first to admit that I did not look "corporate" in terms of the business suits most were wearing and what was known in the '60s, '70s, and '80s as the corporate haircut. A boss once told me my hairstyle suggested I had just gotten out of bed and he found it very distracting. At first we laughed, then we argued about his comment. As would often happen during discussions like this one, he dismissed it by saying that I had taken his comments too personally; after all, he was only kidding. I loved soft feminine clothes and I loved leather. I wore mini skirts and tops that were tight enough to be a second skin. I wore every style during my career. My son would tell you I wore ripped jeans years before Cher made them a fashion statement. I did purchase one three-piece grey suit in a short-lived attempt to dress "like the boys" but it definitely was not me. I personally think you should dress exactly as you please as long as you understand and accept that what you wear does send a message. Eventually I began to "get the message."

One of my most memorable experiences in Ottawa was working with my first female boss. Janis Fawn arrived in Ottawa just after I had promoted one of my employees, Jackie MacKercher. Several of my peers did not support Jackie's promotion to management; they believed I'd promoted her because she was a woman, and their man was a better match for the job. Behind my back they collectively went to Janis and complained about my judgement. When Janis came to me I was hearing the complaint for the first time. I asked Janis to observe Jackie at work and assured her that she too would be supportive of Jackie, and she was. Janis later told me she was impressed with how I handled this situation. I did not confront my peers but chose to allow them to witness Jackie succeeding in her job. I was learning how to play the corporate game.

Just after Janis arrived she saw Jamie and me in my office early one Sunday so she dropped in to visit. Jamie understood the routine for employees moving from city to city very well and asked my boss if she had "moved on the company plan." They carried on an adult conversation as I proudly observed my son sharing all that he knew about Bell. Janis got to know Jamie very well during these Sunday morning conversations.

Janis was a mentor to me and to several other females at Bell. It was wonderful to be able to confide in her and freely seek her advice. She eventually moved to Toronto and tried to pave the way for females there. We would laugh years later when we realized that we were both victims of the male-only National Club because our boss insisted on holding meetings there. We were allowed in, but only if we entered via the back stairwell. We could not dine in the main dining room but in the lower dining area, which was basically the basement. However, you had to play the game if you wanted to move up, so we went along with it.

When Janis left, I became Jim Nolan's first female subordinate. During Jim's very first day on the job he called me to his office and told me he had been reviewing my file and was concerned that I was Northeast Area's token female. I would have to prove to him that I deserved to be in this job. I wanted to say, "God, if I have to prove one more time that I deserve to be in this position I'm going to . . ." That's where the thought always ended. I wanted to succeed. To Jim's credit he was open about his views and I knew immediately where I stood with him. He knew I wanted to work in Installation and Repair and he educated me about the department. One day he came to my office and said, "If you ever want a job in the plant department, young lady, learn to back your car into your parking spot. I just observed your car nose first in your spot. Don't do that again." I backed my car into my parking spot at work and any other spot from that day forward. When Jamie and I were out and he noticed me backing the car into a spot he would jokingly say, "Is Jim Nolan going to be here, Mom?" Jim wasn't comfortable handing out compliments, but when he transferred me to Toronto in the summer of 1978 he told me, "I only send my best."

The move to Toronto was a difficult one in many ways. It was a lateral move, not a promotion, so there would be no salary increase to offset housing prices in Toronto as compared to Ottawa. And in the office I became known as Bell's country bumpkin (behind my back of course). Not only had I come from Bell's Northeast Area, but I was from Nova Scotia, which apparently was sufficient reason to make fun of my background.

I was now dating a co-worker, Denis Gauthier. Denis came to Toronto to help me find and move into my new condo in Lampton Square. When Jamie arrived in late August, his new home was waiting. We had a third bedroom for the first time and he enjoyed his own TV room where his new friends could come to play.

On my first morning in the new job I met my new boss, Murray Makin, and I was so nervous. He was on the phone and I made the mistake of going into his office anyway. I was impressed to see he had a large glass of juice waiting for me, so I enjoyed it while he completed his phone call. When he hung up someone else came into the office and Murray said, "Ron, have you met Carol Ann Cole? This is her first day on the job." Ron said with a smile, "I don't care who the hell you are — you're drinking my goddamn juice." He and Murray had been in the middle of a meeting when Murray had to take a call, so Ron had left the office. He was joking with me, but I was too nervous to understand that at the time. Not a smooth start to my first day in the big city.

A year after my big move to Toronto, I was offered an Installation and Repair job in London, Ontario. I wanted the position, but not the location. I felt strongly that I should be able to get a similar job in Toronto without relocating my son to London so soon after moving. I refused the job, which sent the message out that I was no longer mobile. Jim Nolan heard this and called to give me advice. I didn't even know I had been labelled not mobile and had no idea the consequences of my actions could be so severe. I talked with my supervisor and clarified that I *was* mobile, but not to London at that time. He replied that if I would not take the job in London I was indeed saying I was not mobile. I was made to understand that Toronto — known as the Metro Machine — would not be giving me a job in the plant department any time soon. If they wanted a female in the job they had women who were already part of their own team to promote. My career definitely stalled. Another lesson learned.

I began to grow accustomed to living in Toronto and realized how far I'd come when my friend Donna came to visit. I showed her my big city, told her all about my job, and she would tell me in detail what was going on in her life. Our friendship was as strong as ever. One day I took her to the

Eaton Centre with a plan to meet her after work. An hour later, I remembered how frightened I had been when I first came to Toronto so I went back to check. Sure enough, she was sitting exactly where I had left her, worried about getting lost if she moved from her seat. She was amazed that Jamie was actually coming downtown to my office on the subway all by himself.

My third bedroom was put to good use when my entire family came to visit as we celebrated Lorraine and Tom's wedding in the summer of 1980. Jamie and I were hosts to the bride and groom who came from Calgary; Mom and Connie from Halifax; and Lois, Natalie, and Dawn Marie from Grande Prairie. We celebrated Christmas in the summertime, dined at Mom's favourite restaurant, and did all the things families do when schedules permit them to cast everything aside and be together. I was definitely not letting my work schedule dictate my life at that time.

Three years had passed since my move to the Toronto offices of Bell and finally I was given the job I longed for. I would be the District Manager of Rouge River Installation and Repair. Charlie Labarge selected me for the job and had to defend his decision to his boss. Toronto's VP had a strong reaction: "Why are you putting her into that job? You know, they're not giving points anymore for putting women in men's jobs." Charlie shared my disgust that it seemed the only time to put women in non-traditional jobs was when it would get you some political points with the boss or others. He told our VP he still operated on the old-fashioned belief that you should hire the best person for the job. I felt so proud when he shared that with me.

Bell's human resources department insisted that certain

forms be filled out because I was a woman in a non-traditional job, but Charlie refused. He made it clear that he would treat me as he treated the guys. At our meetings he would greet me by saying, "So Carol Ann, how are the wife and kids?" He finally did complete some forms, but only because HR insisted.

Not only did I have the job I wanted, I had it in Toronto. I called Donna to share the news and she joked that the Halifax newspaper should run the story with the headline, "Country Bumpkin Does Good."

The first day on the job I went to one of the garages at 7 a.m. so I could meet my new team. It was a cold February morning and I was dressed in typical business office attire, which included my fur coat and high-heeled boots. Some of the men watched me park my car (since it was an unfamiliar car it piqued their interest immediately) and one of them came over to me and introduced himself as Bill.

"Pleased to meet you Bill, I'm Carol Ann Cole," I replied. Bill raised his voice a little for his audience as he turned to me and said, "Oh yeah, so who's Carol Ann Cole?"

I didn't want to give him my title right away because it seemed too impersonal so I said, "Well, I'm joining your team, it's my first day on the job." He looked me up and down and said, "Honey, if you're here to go on a riding exercise, you ain't dressed properly. You need steel-toed boots . . ."

I told him I really was there to meet some of my team and that I was replacing Jim Gallaway. Jim had been the District Manager for some time and I was certain Bill would know who he was. I was wrong. Bill had a larger audience now and was strutting as he continued: "Oh yeah, so who's Jim Gallaway?"

I finally put my arm around him and said, "Bill, listen to me. I am your new District Manager. Today is my first day on your team." Bill swore, turned quickly, and left the building. We were all laughing as he drove out of the yard — probably the only time he would arrive at his first service call for the day ahead of schedule.

I had over 300 people on my Rouge River team and decided I wanted to learn all of their names. This was called a "soft skill" at the time and not considered important, but I felt it was critical to know something about each of my teammates — starting with their names. Barb and Sylvia were my secretaries and Barb prepared and maintained a picture book for me. We called it my "cheat book." Each time I left for the garage, I would look up five faces in my cheat book and then find those people at the garage so I could call them by name. It worked and they appreciated it. Eventually I didn't need to consult the cheat book. I also kept an "incident file" and when a young installer would tell me he had gotten married or bought a home I would make a note of that. At year-end I was able to write a personal comment in every Christmas card we sent out. Barb would address the envelope and I would write the note. I learned later the men and women would actually compare cards and ask, "What did she say in yours?" My handwriting has never been all that good, so sometimes they would bring my notes to work so others could help them read what I had written.

The first meeting I had with my entire management team was held in a local hotel. My managers were nervous and so was I. I knew that many had complained when the announcement of my appointment was made: "Who needs a woman in the job?" "Why give us someone who isn't even from Toronto? She doesn't even know that Toronto is different." The meeting was not going well due to the tension in the room so to lighten things up after the morning break, I began what they thought would be a serious discussion. "Gentlemen, if we are going to work together one thing will have to change." You could see the glances around the room and that "I knew it" look on their faces.

"We will never be able to work together until you learn to put the toilet seat down." They burst into laughter. I was now more human in their eyes and we went on to talk about how they really felt and why. I shared with them that I too was nervous and needed their help to succeed. They were proud and happy to help me learn all about their job, and when I took courses designed for installers, they would help me prepare and then call to see how "we" had done.

One of my repair testers, Ron Barton, was also learning how to work with the new boss. I gave him a poster of an animal with a mouth full of tennis balls. The caption read "You gotta have balls." He was reprimanded for putting the poster on the wall and I was reprimanded for giving it to him. We were off to a great start.

Barb was not only an excellent secretary, but she was becoming a good friend. I called her to my office one day to ask a huge favour. I reminded her that I had never asked her to get me a coffee or run an errand but I did need a favour now. "I need you to come to the president's hockey tournament with me. My guys are in the annual president's tournament and I need to be there." She came with me not once, but many times over the years. We even managed to have our picture taken with the Stanley Cup — we called "Stanley" our date! We couldn't have known the day we first attended a hockey tournament that we would later have something else in common — something much less fun and much more personal.

After a year with this team, I received some very exciting and wonderful news. In two weeks I would begin a new job in Montreal. This promotion to the next level would set me up perfectly for future promotions to reach my goal of a VP job before my fortieth birthday. Or so I thought.

On a personal level Montreal was perfect. My childhood friend, Phyllis White (who was now Phyllis Pedicelli), lived there and we would be able to reconnect after so many years. I called her immediately and she offered Jamie and me a room in their home until we found a place of our own. It was so like Phyllis and so like a Maritimer. We didn't stay with her initially but Jamie often stayed with the Pedicellis when my job took me back to Toronto. Phyllis was an excellent cook and Jamie loved eating there. On the other hand, her children Robbie and Chrissy were thrilled to see me arrive often with Tim Horton's muffins. They only got to eat homemade muffins so *this* was considered a treat in their eyes.

Jamie was thirteen years old and I was eager to make him part of the home selection process once again. He would be going to his dad's soon for the summer. I found the ideal condo for us and he came to Montreal for the weekend to participate in the final decision. The sun shone brightly on Saturday morning when Jamie decided to stay at the Hotel Bonaventure pool and relax. I returned to the hotel and I noticed numerous empty glasses and food trays surrounding him as he soaked up the sun. As I approached him he said, "Can you believe this Mom? Just because you are staying here I can have anything I want!" I went directly to the hotel staff to ask why they allowed this to happen. Didn't they realize my thirteen-year-old did not know he was charging everything to my room? The waiter replied, "No Madam, I think he knew *exactly* what he was doing." His lunch was almost as costly as the hotel room.

Jamie was no longer investing in our real estate purchases. "Do you know I am the only kid in my class who has a mother making him help pay for their house?" he marvelled one day after school. So much for my plan to educate him in the world of real-estate investments. He cashed out.

I met my new boss, Ralph McKay, the first day on the job in Montreal. He selected me based on reputation and a telephone conversation with Murray Makin. A number of my male counterparts had informed me that they were offered the job first but Ralph assured me that was untrue. I call it the testosterone factor — some men want you to think that *you* got the job because *they* turned it down.

I was the Director of Labour Relations and would be negotiating contracts for Bell with the Canadian Telephone Employee's Association. I learned during my two years there that the term "non-management" should never be used. Who wants to be called non-anything? I had, and still have great respect for unions and related associations. One of the most powerful unions in Canada would become an unlikely partner with me later in life.

Good food and fine wine go hand in hand in Montreal. Ralph taught me that good wine does not come with a screw top and my favourite wine is still one that I can only find in Quebec. Jamie and I ate out almost every single night and never at the same restaurant. Although I placed an emphasis on my job promotions, the raise in salary over the years helped in many ways. I was no longer a struggling single mother, but I still kept a tight rein on managing my finances. I never went into debt for anything I purchased, and for the first few promotions never spent any money on myself. My weakness for leather and good clothes got the best of me and I splurged on my first designer suit at Chez Catherine, a boutique in Montreal. It was a camel-coloured ostrich leather suit and for the first time I didn't even hesitate at the $2,500 price tag. It was a far cry from my first goal of owning my own washer and dryer!

Jamie also became James in Montreal — to all but me.

Mom visited with me often and I loved to hear her Acadian French as she spoke with Francophones around us. One Christmas season we were in a lovely restaurant and our waiter recognized Mom's Acadian French because he spoke it as well. They had a lengthy conversation (not about me I hope). I knew that my next move was approaching and it would be back to Toronto. I spoke with Mom about leaving her native Nova Scotia and moving to be closer to me. Her four daughters shared a concern that she not grow old alone; she was approaching her sixty-ninth birthday. She agreed and in 1984 we moved Mom to Scarborough, Ontario, just prior to Jamie and I moving to Toronto for a second time.

Between 1984 and 1989 I had a number of jobs in the Toronto area. All were great jobs where I worked with wonderful people, but they were all at the same level. Then, in 1988, it almost happened. I felt certain I was the perfect candidate for one of the two VP jobs available in Ontario, for which only two of us were in the running. I couldn't lose this time. Could I?

My boss, Mike, was also fairly confident but reminded me nothing would be certain until the president's meeting in Montreal the following week even though I kept badgering him for confirmation. I would not let up until Mike said "Yes, go ahead and celebrate, but remember, nothing is official until next week." On Saturday morning I took every piece of gold I owned to a jewelry store and asked to have a very special bracelet created for me. I wanted a "king's link" design, which would be strong, bold, and different. I thought it would be a constant reminder of how hard I had worked to get to the top. I talked to everyone in my family that weekend, telling them the news and accepting their congratulations. Everyone knew how important this promotion was for me. The weekend passed in a blur, and so did the Monday and Tuesday while I waited for the announcement. Late Tuesday afternoon, Mike called me to his office, shut the door, and sat down. This is it, I thought. He is selecting just the right words to congratulate me. He knows how much I want this job and how long I have waited for it.

"Carol Ann," he began, "I am sorry. They gave the job to someone else. I didn't know there was a third name on the table." I was devastated and began to cry, which made Mike uncomfortable. He suggested I take the rest of the day off. He said all the right things: "Your promotion will come. It's just a matter of time." To say I was a wreck would be putting it mildly. I went to my doctor and for the first time in my life I asked for tranquilizers. My disappointment was overwhelming. Murray called me at home that evening and said, "Don't take this personally. This has nothing to do with you. It has everything to do with who your competition was, and in this case it happened to be a couple of guys." Easy for him to say. Nothing would console me — I would wake up in the middle of the night and write notes to my boss explaining why that promotion should have been mine.

I am embarrassed to say I went AWOL. I disappeared for almost a month. I would not go to work, would not return Mike's calls, and would see no one. Finally Mike insisted I meet him for lunch. When we met he simply said, "Carol Ann, I am going to give you a bit of advice. The decision is yours to make, but I am telling you to get back to work, get your head down, and get busy. This has gone on long enough. I can't cover for you much longer." I had been so concerned with losing the VP job that I didn't stop to consider that my current behaviour could be damaging my entire career. This had been a huge mistake on my part, especially for a female climbing the corporate ladder in a male-dominated environment. It made me look emotional and vulnerable — two characteristics I had fought against showing.

I went back to work as Mike had suggested and he continued to be a great mentor. He knew I was looking for a career outside of Bell, but he also knew my heart belonged to the company. In May 1989 Mike called me at home one evening to tell me that Murray wanted to meet with us very early the next morning. I was working on a special assignment for Murray and, assuming he wanted an interim report, was angry that he had given me so little notice.

Mike and I walked into Murray's office without saying a word to each other. Murray got down to business right away. "There is an opening for a VP job. Terry Mosey is being transferred and I have made a decision about who will replace him." My mind was racing. I wanted to say, "At least you've got the balls to tell me to my face this time." Thank God I didn't.

Murray looked straight at me and said, "I'm giving the job to you, Carol Ann. Welcome to the team and congratulations." I'm not sure I spoke a word. I kept looking from Murray to Mike in disbelief. I shook hands with both of them and mumbled something like, "Thank you Murray. You won't be sorry." His reply was very typical: "I'd better not be sorry."

On May 8, 1989, I would become a vice president. I had reached my goal — albeit three years later than I had planned.

Finally I would be in a position where I could make a difference. I could help our customers and I could offer influence and mentorship to many in the company. I could open doors for others.

When my promotion was announced officially, my office was flooded with messages and flowers. I was overwhelmed with support from my Installation and Repair team from the early '80s, who proudly told everyone they were not surprised to hear the news; after all, they had taught me everything I needed to know about the department. I was extremely touched that they were so proud. I shared many laughs with the women from the business offices with whom I would now be working again. They called to remind me that Terry Mosey was "more handsome" than I was and from a female viewpoint they were not happy to see him leave. I agreed.

Jamie and I went to the executive floor — 10 South — the weekend before my big job began. I was proud to show him my executive office and the perks that came with it. Jamie was impressed with my new office and my new car, but not as impressed as he was with the pop stash in the kitchen.

I could no longer send personal notes to everyone on my team at Christmas; it was now over 3,000 strong. I continued to operate with an open door policy and anyone who wanted to see me knew where to find me. I spent as much of my time out of my office as necessary so I could be with those actually making the company run. I attended more banquets in legion halls and ate more roast beef dinners than I can count.

One member of my team was one of the funniest men I knew, and I encouraged Bell to use him as an in-house come-

dian at our functions. When he wasn't working with us, Mike
Bullard was travelling the country doing standup comedy. I
first met Mike when I was scheduled to spend half a day with
him on the job. As I approached him I saw that he had a new
vehicle so I asked him how he had managed that. Not realizing he was a comedian, I wasn't prepared for his reply:
"Please Miss Cole, I have never had anything new in my life
before. Everything I own is used. Even my wife was married
before." Months later I saw Mike just after he changed jobs
and was supervising mainly a female team. I asked how he
was enjoying the job and he quickly replied, "I'm thinking of
getting my colours done after work and that might help." Mike
had a dream at the time. His dream was to turn his love for
comedy into a full-time gig — who knew he would become
a national celebrity!

Becoming a vice president changed my life in many ways,
good and bad. I worked longer hours and was proud to be a
workaholic. My commitment to Bell was endless. I loved talking
with students about careers at Bell and giving speeches on being
a woman in a non-traditional role. It was so rewarding to speak
on behalf of Bell. I hobnobbed with celebrities at gala events
one night and shared beers with my team on the other.

One of my most memorable encounters was with Pierre
Trudeau. Maybe it was because Mom was such a big fan of
his — she read everything about him and loved to watch him
on television. I first met Trudeau when he was still the prime
minister in the early 1980s. He was having dinner at a Montreal
restaurant where I was meeting with my Bell managers. He
sent a glass of wine to my table, and I went over to thank
him. He was gentle and warm and joked that he was curious
why I was having dinner with so many men. A few years later

I met him again in the same restaurant. He was having dinner with his sons. I approached him this time, reminding him I had met him years earlier. As I told him Bell was now sending me back to Toronto he took my hand and with his trademark charm he said, "Well, I will have to speak with Bell about that now, won't I?" He introduced me to his sons, and was very gracious. A third meeting was at a health spa, but when he saw that I could not keep up with him during an exercise class he moved on to someone else. Mom was thrilled to hear of these chance meetings and would make me repeat everything to her in detail. Each time I spoke with Trudeau, I would send Mom a postcard that read:

> **Mrs. Cole,**
> **You have a lovely daughter.**
> **Signed, Pierre**

My friend Diane Cummings sent me a card when I was promoted that read, "Congratulations, you have become the person your mother wanted you to marry." That may have been true of many mothers, but not mine. My promotion signified the realization of that whispered conversation long ago in Wilmot. I had achieved all that Mom had expected of me and her confidence over the years was unwavering.

I had reached the pinnacle of my life. I had the support of my family and friends. My son was developing into a fine young man, my career goals had been met, and I was secure financially. All the pieces of my life had come together and I was now prepared to enjoy them. Little did I know how much I would come to relish every one of those aspects in the coming year.

The Cancer Arena

$\mathcal{T}$he balmy breezes off the ocean should have been a solace to someone who had just flown in from a Canadian winter. I had come to the Dominican Republic with my friend Valerie for a few days of rest and relaxation before starting the new year. Valerie and I had decided at the last minute to fly down because we didn't have any plans to celebrate New Year's Eve. But the hot weather, beautiful resort, and relaxed atmosphere could not lessen my feeling of dread. I had a lump in my breast. Throughout the four days we were on vacation, my hand would stray across my chest. I could cross my arms and my fingertips would just graze the lump. One moment I could find it, and another I would think, *Oh it could be anything*. I had looked at myself naked in front of the mirror that morning, and couldn't see anything out of the ordinary. I tried not to think of the "C" word, and believed if it really were cancerous, it would be more noticeable.

Until now I have told people that I found the lump myself. That is not true. A man I had just begun dating found it. Brian and I had known each other for a few years. We lived in the same neighbourhood and both worked out daily at Gold's Gym. The extent of our conversations was, for the most part, small talk, but there was a great chemistry between the two of us and I could feel it the moment we started talking. So I was flattered and excited when we had our first date on Boxing Day in 1991. Brian was a massage therapist, making us an unlikely couple — me with my briefcase and Brian with his massage oil. Our first date was very special and we ended up back at my apartment. Since we had been attracted to each other for so long, things escalated quite quickly and we became intimate. That's when Brian felt the lump in my breast. He was concerned and we talked about it; Brian wanted me to go to the doctor immediately.

I wanted to believe "it was nothing," and given the time of year I felt certain it would be difficult to see my doctor until after the new year. So with trepidation, I went on vacation instead. I spent much of the time going for walks on the beach and reading. I was less social than I normally would have been, since I was emotionally troubled by what would possibly happen to me. As I dressed for a New Year's Eve party, I wondered if I would be able to wear a similar dress in the future. Would I lose my breast?

When I returned from the Dominican Republic, I wasn't convinced the lump was cancerous, but I was worried. Brian had flooded my answering machine with phone calls, setting up appointments for me and encouraging me to get to a doctor as quickly as possible. I saw my doctor on January 3 and he told me I needed to see a cancer specialist immediately. I reminded him I had had a mammogram two months earlier and nothing showed up. He called Doctor Saul Sidlofsky at Mount Sinai Hospital with me listening to the conversation. He explained that I needed to see the doctor urgently (he obviously felt something I hadn't when he checked the lump). I was struck by the seriousness in his voice as he asked me to let him know how things went at my appointment on January 15. I left his office worried that cancer had knocked on my door.

I didn't want to tell any of my family until I knew for certain if the lump was cancerous. There was a history of cancer in our family, and I knew that if I told Mom she would worry. Even though she was now living nearby, I found it difficult to even think about visiting her. I was afraid I might say something about the lump before I was ready to share my news with her. I thought a lot about Brian — he was a man with whom I had wanted to connect for a long time. I really thought he might be my life partner. I didn't want to burden him with what was happening to me, especially after only one date. Despite my reservations, Brian and I spent much of the next few days together. I was very preoccupied with the looming appointment and tried to ensure things were in order at work "just in case." I tried to carry on as usual, which meant priority one was my job. En route to a meeting at one of my repair bureaus, I called my boss to tell him that I had a doctor's appointment coming up and it might result in needing some time off work. I felt too emotional to discuss it in person, so I did it over the phone, telling Murray about the lump in my breast and the history of breast cancer in my family without having to face him.

A few days later, on January 8, I received a call that changed my life. I returned to my office just after 5 p.m., having been out with my installation team for the day. My phone was ringing as I entered the office. I was still in my workboots and hadn't even removed my coat as I grabbed the phone. My mom was on the line, which was very unusual; she rarely called me at work. She had joked over the years about never disturbing me at my "big job."

"Hey Mom, what's up?"

"Carol Ann, I need you to come right away, I just found out I have breast cancer," she said in a whisper.

As I held the receiver in my hand, I am sure I went into shock. The first thing that flashed through my mind was that someone had told my mother I had a lump in my breast. How else could she know? Is it possible she is talking about me — not herself? I was very confused and could only say, "Mom, what are you talking about?" She told me she had been to the doctor that day and he had confirmed that she had breast cancer. She was scheduled to be admitted to the hospital the next day to await surgery. I will never forget the tone in her voice as she said, "Carol Ann, I need you to come right away. I need your support."

I snapped out of my confusion and told Mom I would rush to my car and call her from the cell phone. That way we wouldn't lose another second. We could talk as I drove to her. To this day I do not remember the actual drive up the DVP to Mom's home in Scarborough. My thoughts were racing from the lump in my breast to how I would tell my mother to what was going to happen to both of us. For an instant I thought about my job. I called my boss and told him my mother had been diagnosed with cancer. I'm sure he thought I was losing my mind; a few days earlier I had told him of the lump in my breast and now I was telling him my mother had cancer. Of course, it never occurred to me to forget work. The next morning I was scheduled to kick off a conference with my entire management team and I assured my boss I would be there. He asked me to keep him informed and I hung up and called my mom. All we focused on during the conversation was how our family would deal with this diagnosis. The first thing Mom wanted to do was call my sisters — she was always concerned about treating the four of us as equals and since I now knew, she would want to call them right away. We were talking about whether or not they should all come home before the surgery as I parked the car. I told Mom I would be up in a minute, hung up the phone, and turned the engine off. I could hardly make my legs move as I got out of the car.

Our routine when I went to Mom's place would be for her to buzz me in and then stand in her doorway peeking out of her apartment to watch me get off the elevator. We would laugh and chat as I walked down the hall. Not this time. Her door remained closed as I approached. I knocked softly and opened the door. Mom was sitting in her favourite chair. She looked half her size, almost as if she had sunken into herself. It was an image that has stuck in my mind forever. She looked at me and said, "Oh Carol Ann," and we both started to cry.

We called my three sisters, one by one, and Mom shared her frightening news. It was a very difficult conversation for Mom to have and for me to listen to. She asked each of them if they would be able to come to Scarborough. We made plans for flights and decided who would come now versus later. Since Lois could not take the time off work right away, she and Mom decided it would be better for her to come during Mom's recovery period. Connie would fly in from Hawaii and Lorraine would come from Calgary the next day. After calling "her girls," Mom and I discussed plans to take her to Scarborough General Hospital the next day. Then Mom asked me to leave — she was always able to compartmentalize her emotions very quickly. There were things she needed to prepare before the surgery and she wanted some time alone. She had a list of items to pack and chores to do. I felt odd leaving Mom alone the evening before she would be going into the hospital, but that was the way she wanted it to be. I knew from years of experience that when Mom decided on something, it was a waste of time to try to change her mind.

I drove back to my apartment and immediately called each of my sisters again, needing to talk to them. The tears were flowing as we discussed the fact that Mom's cancer may be very advanced. It was incomprehensible to us that she had kept it a secret for so long. A year ago we had celebrated her seventy-fifth birthday with a huge party. It was an exciting day for her. In her diary she had written that it was one of the happiest times:

> My 75th birthday party — 4 p.m. at Carol Ann's. This evening was the happiest time for me. I never thought on my 75th birthday I would be so lucky. So many lovely gifts, all my friends and my family. I could never put into words how I feel tonight. Lois, Carol Ann, Lorraine, and Connie I love you all so very much. Oh, it's midnight, I'm happy and so tired. Good night.

Mom looked like the healthiest person alive at her party and the photographs confirm it. As my sisters and I talked, we realized that she must have had cancer even then. Mom had lost siblings to cancer and it seemed many in her family had had a brush with it at some point in their lives. I'm sure it terrified her that she might be next, and she chose to ignore the possibility of it happening to her. Looking back in her diaries, I later found her entry on New Year's Day, 1992: "I would like to write here what I want for this year, but I cannot do it. I'm only hoping for the impossible." Who could have known that as mom wrote about her fears in her diary, I would be contemplating the same thing about myself while on vacation in the Dominican Republic.

After talking with each of my sisters and telling Connie and Lorraine I would meet them at the hospital the next day, I called Mom. She was getting ready for bed and I quickly sensed she wanted to be alone with her thoughts. I promised I would be there early in the morning, but didn't tell her I would first be at a conference. Next I called one of my managers and told him about my family emergency. I assured him I would arrive at the hotel early the next morning to kick off the conference, but that I would have to leave immediately after. It didn't enter my mind not to go — Bell was part of who I was.

The next morning I was up very early and drove to the hotel for the breakfast meeting. I checked into the hotel where my sisters and I could be together the night before Mom went into surgery. I met first with the nine managers who worked directly with me and told them about Mom having cancer and me having to leave the conference right away. I did not mention the lump in my breast; at this point I was only concerned about my mother. I reminded them I would turn the conference over to them. I could tell they were worried about me giving the opening address, but I assured them I was under control emotionally. I went to the podium and introduced the guest speaker, explaining to the assembled group that there would be a change in plans. "This is a very difficult morning for me," I began. "I just found out last evening that my mom has cancer." At that point I started to cry uncontrollably. I could see my managers looking stricken as I left the stage as fast as I could. I raced to the car and to my mother.

When I picked Mom up the tears were still rolling down my face, and I continued to cry all the way to the hospital. She was admitted immediately. Not long after she was settled in bed, Lorraine arrived and began to take charge. Lorraine's husband Tom was a doctor and had made several calls already to ensure Mom was receiving the best care and treatment possible. Tom's knowledge combined with Lorraine's nursing expertise put my sisters and me at ease, and we were happy to take a back seat at this stage. Mom was very nervous, anxious, and quiet. Connie arrived and Mom was grateful that she had come all the way from Hawaii within twenty-four hours. Lorraine and I went for a walk to allow Mom some private time with "her baby." Additional tests were completed and in the evening, after Mom had fallen asleep, we joined the doctors for a medical briefing. Thank God Lorraine was with us; I wasn't sure I could understand any of it.

I had told my sisters about finding the lump in my breast, but now was not the time to talk about it. I worried that if I spoke about my problem, it would draw attention away from Mom. I had also mentioned it to Mom as casually as I could, and assured her I had already been to the doctor to have it checked out. I did not want her to worry, but thought I should mention it just in case she later wondered why I had not told her earlier.

As we sat in a conference room listening to an outline of

the impending surgery and Mom's condition, I felt like I was having an out-of-body experience. The bright overhead lights and hard chairs all disappeared as soon as I heard the discussion turn to the lumps in Mom's breast. The doctors were using a blackboard to help us understand the next day's operation. They had drawn a breast on the board with the tumour. As they talked about the size and thickness of the tumour, my fingers would touch the lump in my breast. I would relate everything they said back to my own tumour and a sense of alarm washed over me. I fought this sensation by telling myself to get over it; this was clearly about Mom and not about me. Yet a little voice in my head would not rationally listen. I snapped out of it long enough to hear one doctor say the cancer had spread to Mom's other breast as well. They would have to perform a full mastectomy on the right breast and a partial mastectomy on the left. The worst was yet to come as the doctor explained his fear that the cancer had spread throughout her body. Connie and I let Lorraine ask all the questions and weigh all the answers, and we looked to her for assurance that everything was being done as it should be.

We said goodnight to Mom and went to the hotel where I was holding my conference. On the way to our room we met some of my managers and I could see the concern on their faces. I left Connie and Lorraine in the room and went downstairs to join my team for a drink. I'm sure my sisters thought I was crazy to do this at such an emotional time, but my career was so intertwined with my personal life at the time that it was just natural for me to do this. I had to make sure my team could see I was okay. We talked about how the conference had gone that day, what was on the agenda for the next morning and they asked about Mom. Some of the men began to share their own cancer stories, but I just wasn't ready to hear them — it was too close and personal.

Early the next morning we returned to the hospital to be with Mom before she went into surgery. We waited anxiously for three hours before the doctor came out and told us the surgery had gone very well. That was the good news. The bad news was that our mother was very ill; the cancer had indeed spread. He told us Mom would not recover, and the only thing we could do was make her as comfortable as possible. "She will have good days and bad days," he told us gently. Mom had instructed us that Lorraine was to see her first when she returned to her room. As the family nurse, Lorraine would help mom "get fixed up" before Connie and I entered the room. It was so emotional when we first saw her. Mom was so tiny and frail, but she had a smile on her face as she shared with us how relieved she was to have survived the surgery.

Mom wanted all the details of the surgery. We had to tell her that while the surgery had been successful, they were unable to remove all of the cancer — it was still in her body. That night she wrote in her diary that she would try to make the best of it while she could:

Today my life was changed forever. I have cancer. On this morning I had surgery. From this day on whatever will happen I don't know, only God knows. But I can live with it, sunshine or darkness. I will make the best of it. I can do it. My heart is filled with love for you girls, God bless you always Lois, Carol Ann, Lorraine, and Connie. I don't know how to thank you and I didn't mean to upset your life.

The next day Mom was up and walking through the corridors with our help. We walked up and down those halls for five days, encouraging Mom and laughing about old times. When my sisters and I were together we always seemed to laugh a lot and carry on, more so this time with the relief of the surgery behind us. Mom would tell us to be quiet, that we were embarrassing her because we were so loud, but she always had a smile on her face as she said it. Mom would constantly remind us to call Lois so that she knew what was going on and wouldn't feel left out. There was a TV show called *Sisters* on at the time and the nurses told us we reminded them of the characters on that show.

I called my friend Donna from a pay phone at the hospital to tell her about Mom's cancer, the lump in my breast, and my impending appointment with the cancer specialist. We cried together and the moments of silence between us made me realize how much Donna understood me as a friend.

This situation was all very difficult for Jamie to understand and accept. By this time he was a young man of twenty, living in Barrie and fulfilling his dreams in the ski world. Despite the distance, he drove down almost every day to visit his grandmother. He was very close to her and had enjoyed many wonderful times with her during his young life. To see her in the hospital bed was very difficult for him. Because we shared everything I had told him immediately about the lump in my breast. I tried to stay positive about it and kept assuring him I would probably not be facing the same situation his grandmother was in.

One day when he had been visiting Mom in the hospital, he asked me to walk him to his car. We walked through the hospital lobby arm-in-arm, our shoulders slumped and our faces stained with tears. Finally Jamie whispered, "What will I do if this happens to you? What happens if this is not only about Grandmother?" We were both so frightened and at that moment I had no answers. Usually I could answer any question he might have, but this was not one of those times.

Five days after Mom had surgery, I visited Dr. Sidlofsky for a needle biopsy. I knew the test would involve inserting a needle into the lump in my breast and drawing fluid, which was then used to determine if the lump was cancerous. Connie came with me and Lorraine stayed with Mom in the hospital.

After Dr. Sidlofsky finished the procedure, he advised me it would take some time for him to receive the test results and he would call me when they were available. He told me he would not know if I had cancer until the test results were available.

"My mother just had surgery for breast cancer on January 10," I blurted out, "and I am so frightened."

He looked at the calendar on his desk and said, "You mean January last year, not last Friday, right?" And then he looked at me with a very serious look on his face. "You don't mean a few days ago, do you?"

"I mean last Friday," I cried.

He stared at me for a moment, reached over to pat my arm and said, "It would be horrible for you to have to go through this at the same time as your mom. We'll find out and we'll get back to you as soon as we can." I left his office and went into the waiting room where Connie was sitting. We burst into tears the instant we saw each other. We didn't want to believe it, but in our hearts we already knew.

I was in denial. I simply *couldn't* have cancer. I was very fit. I went to the gym every day at 6 a.m. for God's sake! Fitness had always been a regular part of my life and my workouts were sacred. Even if I was facing a long day at work, I always went to the gym — not only did it reduce stress, but it also helped me mentally prepare for each day. I didn't look like I had cancer, did I?

During my career I was always too busy working to celebrate. I would put everything important to me on hold, or save it in what I called my pending file until I could take time to enjoy it. When someone would suggest they had an interesting man to introduce me to, I would say, "Put him in my pending file for now." The day we brought Mom home from the hospital, all that changed. We were taking the time to celebrate having her home, being together, and enjoying dinner. Mom looked radiant as we sat around the table. We held hands and she told us how much she loved us. I am not sure Mom had ever openly told me she loved me before; not in words, anyway.

It was a bittersweet evening for me. We were still awaiting my test results. When we returned to my home, I discovered two messages from Dr. Sidlofsky's office on my answering machine. The first was a regular message asking me to return their call when I had time. Connie rubbed my shoulders as I listened to the second message.

"Carol Ann, this is Doctor Sidlofsky. Call me at this number as soon as you get in. It's very important." My hands trembled as I dialed his number and I looked into Connie's eyes as Doctor Sidlofsky confirmed my worst fears.

"Carol Ann, you have breast cancer."

Half Past Cancer

After talking with Dr. Sidlofsky, a feeling of absolute fear washed over me. Even though I had thought about cancer constantly since Mom's call to me at the office, it was now a reality. Cancer was going to kill my mother and I had it too. At the same time I was forcing myself to stay positive — I was convinced that since the lump hadn't been there for very long, the cancer could not be that advanced. The mammogram would have detected a cancerous lump, wouldn't it? I told myself I would have the surgery and then do everything it took to beat it. "I'll take time off work and just focus on recovery. I'll put my big job at the Bell in my pending file — I promise!"

I was scheduled to have surgery on January 27, a week and a half away. It seemed like a long time to wait, but there was much to do in the meantime. While it was hard to accept the diagnosis, I knew I had to call everyone who had been waiting just as anxiously for the test results. I called Jamie first to tell him the news — we talked for a very long time and cried together. He shared my positive attitude and we knew we would beat it together. I called Lois and cried again. It was hard for Lois to be away from us during this terrible time, but we looked forward to her visit when we were on the road to recovery. My next call was to Lorraine and Mom. After I told Lorraine, she put Mom on the phone, and we spoke briefly. Lorraine told me later that Mom was crying when she hung up, and she had said to my sister, "I think I'll just go to bed now. Good night, Lorraine." Giving my mother the news was one of the hardest things I have ever had to do. It must be so difficult for any parent to be told their child has cancer and for Mom, this diagnosis was so close to her own. Tears were running down my face as I picked up the phone to call Brian. I told him I had cancer, and then tried to find the right words to let him know I would understand if he wanted to back off from the relationship. We had only been dating a few weeks and I did not want him to feel he had to be by my side. Brian was very concerned and confessed he hated hospitals and definitely would not visit me there. I got the sense that he wanted some space, but understood how he felt; dealing with cancer can put stress on any relationship, not just a new one.

Connie had been standing beside me through all the phone calls, and had shared my tears. We also shared a bottle of wine as we talked about the upcoming surgery and what had to be done before the date. When I told her I really had cried enough and was calm enough to call my boss, she looked at me in shock.

"Are you sure you want to make that call?" she asked. "You can tell me what to say and I can call him for you." Connie was always amazed at the loyalty I felt towards the company. I called Murray and started to cry as soon as I told him about being diagnosed with cancer. He talked with me about my diagnosis for a long time before the talk turned to work. I saw a softer side of Murray that most never see. He asked what would be the most comfortable way to tell my co-workers at Bell. We agreed that I would send an e-mail to my team and he would inform my peers and the rest of the executive team.

That night I sat down in front of my computer for a long time before I could find the right words. I forwarded a very personal note to at least 300 people, asking them to share the message with everyone else on my team. I apologized for not being totally honest with them at the conference and explained why I had handled it that way. I told them I would have to be away for a while, but assured them I would be at the Blue Jays' home opener in April with many of them. I was trying to make sure they knew this was only a temporary thing and I would be back working with them soon.

The day after I sent the message my phone began ringing off the hook. It seemed everyone wanted to talk to me before the surgery, and I tried to reassure them that I would be okay. Connie was upset with all the phone calls. "What's wrong with this picture?" she would fume as I took another call from someone at Bell. It upset her to see me spending this critical time before the surgery comforting other people. Connie joked that she was going to have the hospital put a security guard by my door and ask anyone who came to see me if they had Bell I.D. If they did, they wouldn't be admitted!

I thought the week before surgery would be a long one, but it passed very quickly. I spent several mornings at Mount Sinai hospital undergoing different tests, and during the afternoons Connie and I would drive to Scarborough to visit Mom and Lorraine. As soon as my diagnosis had been confirmed, Connie decided to stay with us for another month. I was grateful for her company. Connie was my best friend as well as my youngest sister and I drew strength from her. She found it hard to watch me going through this, but she could always make me laugh.

I was very nervous about my upcoming operation, but I tried hard to put on a different face in front of Mom. I could see how concerned she was about me every time I looked into her eyes and it broke my heart. We all tried to focus on Mom and helping her feel better. Mom was doing her exercises and I took pleasure in instructing her — I had never seen Mom exercise!

In that last week before surgery I struggled to follow my regular routine. I drew energy going to the gym and went daily. I wondered if I would be able to wear my work-out tank tops after my surgery; I purchased a few high neck tops just in case. Lingering fears and doubts kept creeping into my mind.

I have always said that Jamie and I had grown up together. Cancer brought our relationship to a different level. Jamie drove down from Barrie every day that week and we talked about his grandmother, his girlfriend Tracey, and my cancer. He wondered if he should move home during my recovery, but I assured him that Connie was with me and he should not disrupt his life to that extent. One day his buddy Howie came with him and I observed that Howie was treating Jamie a little differently than he usually did. I mentioned it to Jamie and he had noticed it, too. His friends were trying so hard to help him through this but — like motherhood — cancer doesn't come with a manual.

When Jamie left after those visits, I began to question my mothering skills. I was being hit with the realization of my own mortality, and I worried that maybe I had not spent enough time with Jamie during all those years I had been working late at the office. For the first time I was beginning to wonder if I had done the right thing by giving my career such a high priority. I had never doubted these decisions before, but the cancer diagnosis made me re-evaluate what was significant in my life. I could only hope it was not too late to change. Whenever someone called from Bell, regardless of their good wishes, the talk would always turn to problems at work. In a joking tone I would say, "Listen to me — I don't care." I knew I had to refocus my energy and concentrate on beating cancer, not solving a problem at work.

As I prepared to go to the hospital the day before my surgery, my neighbours, Rosemary and John Teed, arrived at my door with breakfast served on a beautiful antique tray. They offered to drive me to the hospital but I was adamant that I would walk instead. Connie and I walked down Yonge Street, and we joked that she carried my luggage and I carried my cancer. I needed to observe life as it was unfolding around me. It was a Sunday and Yonge Street was busy with people strolling with a coffee in hand or window-shopping. We cried as we entered Mount Sinai Hospital on University Avenue, unsure of what tomorrow would bring.

All of the vibrant activity on the street was in stark contrast to the quiet halls of the hospital. As soon as I began the check-in process, I was overwhelmed with anxiety. I felt vulnerable and nauseous about what was going to happen during the surgery. The nurse told me I had lost thirteen pounds in the week since my mother's surgery, and it made me feel very frail. I thought I would have some time to think once I got settled in my room, but Mount Sinai is a teaching hospital, and many of the doctors brought their students in to see me. I may have been considered an interesting case, since my mother had been operated on a week earlier, and I was kept very busy answering questions. One of the doctors came in to have me sign the papers for my surgery, and I noticed the chart said I was having a mastectomy. I wanted the doctor to change it, so he added "partial" in front of the word mastectomy, but that would not satisfy me. I wanted to see the word "lumpectomy" because that was what I was having. I did not want to see the word mastectomy anywhere on the page. I needed to feel in control of the situation and was nervous about the whole procedure. The doctor finally did change it, re-typing the form, and I felt more comfortable.

When I shared this story with Barb, she told me — for the first time — that I had done something similar to her when we first worked together in Rouge River Installation and Repair. The very first letter she typed up for me had one word I wanted changed, so I stroked through the entire letter rather than pointing out the one small change to her. This was in the days before computers and correcting tape. She was not amused.

Connie and Jamie were with me the night before the surgery, and I talked to Mom and Lorraine at home before I went to bed. I wanted to reassure Mom that everything would be okay, and I told her I would call again after the surgery the next day. It was hard to believe that just weeks before I had been on the opposite side of the hospital bed as we awaited Mom's surgery. In her diary the next day Mom wrote about her fears that she couldn't voice:

Today Carol Ann is being operated on for cancer. I just can't put the words here how I feel today. Please make her well and fill her life with happiness. Always she's helping others, now she needs so much support.

Early the next morning, Connie and Jamie came back to be with me before the operation. We were very quiet — they were reassuring me that they would be there as soon as I woke up. My last memory before surgery was of Connie and Jamie walking beside the gurney to the operating room. They later told me that as they walked back to the elevator, the doors opened and a big guy came running out. Jamie looked at him and said, "Let me guess, you're Brian. You're too late." Brian looked at him in shock, thinking something had happened to me. Jamie explained he was too late to see me. I had already gone into surgery. I had not heard from Brian that week and assumed he had decided to back away from the relationship.

When I awoke from surgery, Jamie and Connie were standing on either side of my bed. I was pleasantly surprised to see Brian at the foot of my bed, massaging my feet. Obviously he had had a change of heart. It made me feel very comfortable to have all of them with me. The surgeon came to talk with me shortly after. I asked immediately if they had gotten all the cancer and he said he was hopeful. A very small incision was required to do the lumpectomy, but they had also removed thirteen lymph nodes, which worried all of us. I thought something was wrong if they had to remove so many. They had sent tissue samples to pathology, so the doctor wouldn't know for certain if everything was okay until he got the reports back. It was almost unbearable waiting for the final answer from pathology.

Later that evening, I called Mom. It was a very emotional phone call as she told me she understood the surgery had gone better for me than her. I know she was comparing her outcome to what mine would be, and I reassured her everything was going to be okay — even though I still didn't know if the cancer was totally gone.

I received so many visitors and phone calls during my time in the hospital, despite the fact that Connie was checking for Bell I.D.! One of my close friends from Bell, Teri McDowell, came to the nurse's station the first night. It was very late and I could hear her talking to the nurse. She had brought me candy and flowers but didn't want to disturb me. I heard the anxious tone in her voice as she questioned the nurse. She softly said, "I know what you are saying, but is she going to be okay? I need her to be okay." Another of my friends, Anne Jenkins, continued a tradition that we had started years earlier. Whenever one of us was sick, the other would bring slippers. This tradition had seen us through some hard times. Although we hadn't seen each other in a few years, the slippers arrived shortly after my surgery. I enjoyed all the visits, even though I was very weak and had difficulty staying awake.

I was only in the hospital for a few days and was sent home before the pathology results arrived. Connie and Brian took me home, and when we arrived at the condo the concierge was loading dozens of floral arrangements on a huge dolly. It took several trips to bring them all to my ninth-floor condo. Connie told me that she had suggested to everyone that they send their good wishes to my home rather than to the hospital. It was wonderful to see all those flowers and to know how many people cared. But, honestly, it became a bit of a joke as they continued to arrive daily. People going through the lobby were beginning to think I had died! One day, the executive vice president at Bell, Jack Sinclair, sent three long-stemmed yellow roses by limousine. Connie came into the bedroom with the three roses in a vase and laughed, "I don't know who this Jack guy is, but if he didn't spend all his money on limousines, he could have sent a lot more than three roses!"

It was great to have Connie with me as I recovered at home — she always knew when to make me laugh. As soon as I got home I was eager to show her my incisions. Her reply was, "*These* little incisions are what all this fuss is about?" We laughed for hours. I wasn't able to see Mom, since we were both supposed to be in our homes recuperating from the surgery. At first I travelled back to the hospital daily because of a few minor complications. I had a great deal of pain in my arm where the lymph nodes had been removed. I would later learn this is a huge problem for many women following breast cancer surgery. Brian would take me to the hospital every day and then back home where he would give me a massage to ease the pain.

Other than family and Brian, Karen Hickey was the first friend to visit me at home following my surgery. She called to insist that while she knew I was not well and did not feel like having any visitors she urgently needed to see me. It had to be that very day. I agreed to her visit, but reminded her that seeing me wouldn't be "pretty" and that she should expect the worst. In she pranced, dressed to the nines in a brand new outfit from one of our favourite stores in Yorkville, fresh from the hairdresser and looking like she was about to go to Hollywood. Seeing just how bad I looked she then burst out laughing and said, "I absolutely *knew* I would look better than you today so here I am. This is payback time for the day you told the sales clerk in Montreal that you should not have to pay as much for a pair of leather pants as I did because, after all, your pants would require less than half the leather mine would take." We laughed so hard I had to force myself to stop because my incisions were hurting!

A week after surgery, my oncologist Dr. Martin Blackstein called and asked me to come in for the pathology results. Connie and Brian came with me, even though I was determined to get the results by myself. I was trying to toughen myself up again, but as I sat in the doctor's office, I felt faint. What if they hadn't gotten all of the cancer? What if I had to undergo chemotherapy?

A great sense of relief washed over me when Dr. Blackstein came in and quickly said, "You are a very lucky lady." He told me the cancer had been self-contained in the one tumour and all the lymph nodes they had removed were free of cancer as well. Dr. Blackstein suggested radiation treatments and prescribed tamoxifen for me to start taking immediately. Lorraine had done some research for me on the drug and although she had some reservations, I made the decision to begin taking it right away.

Dr. Blackstein explained there would be a wait to start radiation, and I was concerned about not being able to begin right away. The waiting list was so long that it would be the end of March or early April before I could have my first radiation treatment, which conflicted with my plans to return to work in March. But I realized the radiation was the most important thing, and that I was so lucky not to require anything worse. I left the hospital that day with much more optimism than I had had during the weeks following Mom's surgery; the news had given me my "anything is possible" attitude back.

The period before Mom and I began radiation treatments was one of reflection and recovery. As a family, we began to deal with everything that had happened in the past month. We not only grieved for what we had been through, we focused on what we would need to do in the coming months. I finally gave in to the exhaustion I had been feeling from the surgery and took some time to relax. I thought a lot about what both Mom and I had been through and what we would now endure. For a time I was very angry that cancer had hit Mom so hard — she was healthy and fit and always looked after everybody else. Her faith in her church and God had not prevented her from getting cancer, and I struggled to find a reason why it had happened to her. I came to the conclusion that we were diagnosed at the same time for a reason. Maybe God made sure we went through cancer together so we could support each other. There is a black humour that exists between cancer survivors and we were there for each other during happy and sad days. There would be plenty of both.

At the end of February, Lorraine and Connie had to go back to their own families and their own lives. Lois arrived and Mom was very excited to have her home for a month. On February 28 Mom wrote in her diary:

Today Lois came home for a month. It will be good for Carol Ann and I to have her here. We will need support and cheering up during our treatments and to go on with our lives.

I met my boss in early February for lunch. I had to tell Murray that I would not be coming back to work any time soon. I would be starting radiation treatments late in March and didn't feel strong enough to deal with work on top of Mom's situation and my own. Murray understood completely. He told me I looked much better than he thought I would, and wondered if I would like to drop by an upcoming conference so everyone could see me. He said my co-workers were very worried about me and he thought they would feel much better if they could see me. I liked the idea and agreed to go, but I immediately went shopping for an outfit that would make me look heavier. I had lost a lot of weight and I worried everyone would see that as a sign of sickness. I selected a bright orange ultra-suede suit with big shoulder pads and a long skirt. I felt confident as I entered the conference room for a brief appearance. In that short time I was able to reassure everyone that I was going to get better. It was the first time I realized how comfortable I was talking about my illness and how easy it was to listen to other people's stories about cancer. It was a completely different experience than when I'd been speaking to my co-workers the evening of Mom's surgery. I wouldn't be returning to work for a few months, but Murray had done me a huge favour when he suggested I attend that conference.

Mom and I began our radiation treatments in April — hers at Sunnybrook Hospital and mine at Princess Margaret Hospital. Once we started our treatments, it filled up most of our time and pretty much became our life. We were a mother-and-daughter team caught in the cancer web. In the mornings I would go for my radiation treatment and then pick Mom up and take her to Sunnybrook for hers. Mom was so tiny and I always had this vision of her under a great big machine, so I waited right outside of the room where she had her radiation. My doctor's notes at the time always said I seemed incredibly fatigued, which was inevitable with all that was going on in our lives. But I also cherished the time I spent with her — we had a lot of down days during this period, but we also had good days.

We tried to stay positive, but would also allow ourselves "pity parties" if the need arose. Brian had forbidden me to eat fast food during the radiation treatment period, but every Friday Mom and I would drive to McDonald's for lunch. We would even drive out of town so we wouldn't be caught and we shared so many laughs. We would eat hamburgers, fries, and ice cream, while observing everyone around us. One day Mom turned to me and said, "I bet we are the only people in this restaurant who have been zapped more than the food." We would sit in these restaurants for hours. If someone looked as if they were complaining a great deal, Mom would say, "Let's invite them over here and see what they really have to complain about."

We were able to help each other so much, and could almost feel what the other was thinking or needing. Hope for us at that time came in many ways: a reassuring smile for each other, lending an arm for Mom to lean on, and she giving me her shoulder to cry on when it all seemed too much. Mom's joy in life, her spirit, and her energy had always been my inspiration. As I watched Mom struggle at her age to be more open with her emotions, I learned how to do the same. I was no longer shy about telling Jamie or my sisters how much I loved them every time we spoke.

One soggy rainy day when I finished my radiation treatment I was angry to see that someone had stolen my raincoat. I talked of nothing else as I drove Mom to Sunnybrook. When she finished her treatment and observed that her coat was still there she said, "Well, I guess my coat isn't even good enough for someone to steal. Let's take some money from that big job at the Bell of yours and buy two new raincoats!" She suggested to me that perhaps someone had taken my coat in error, or perhaps it had been stolen by someone who needed it more than I. Another lesson learned.

Although I took Mom to almost all of her radiation treatments, there were two days where I was just too weak to be with her. The first time I had a friend pick Mom up, and she called me as soon as she got home from her treatment. She wanted to know if I was okay, and refused to talk about her own treatment. She would always say to me, "Carol Ann, you know this is too much for you. You shouldn't be doing this." I didn't want her to be more concerned about me than herself. Ross Strain, one of my managers at Bell, sent me a note saying he had lined up rides to pick Mom up if ever I should need help from my friends at work. The note listed the day and the driver available to help us — all I had to do was call. I was always touched that many of my friends at Bell didn't just make the offer to help, but had a plan to make it happen.

My sisters and I knew that our time with Mom was limited, and we made sure her wishes were being carried out. As soon as we finished our radiation treatments, Mom made her list of things she wanted to see and the trips began.

First, Lorraine and I took Mom to Niagara-on-the-Lake. Mom loved it there. During our stay Lorraine was helping Mom with her exercises when Mom asked if I would like to see her scars. It broke my heart. Later, when Mom and I were alone she sometimes talked about how she felt about having lost her breast. Even at Mom's age of seventy-six, she felt very unattractive and would comment on how "ugly" she felt at certain times. Many women never get over the emotional strain of breast cancer.

Next Mom and I travelled to Ottawa for a weekend. Mom was tired after the long drive and she needed a day of rest before we could execute her plan. She was determined to tour the Parliament Buildings one last time, and I told her, "If I have to go to the Parliament Buildings with you again, you are coming to see the movie *Sister Act* with me." We did both and Mom loved the movie — it was the last film we saw together.

Mom clearly enjoyed the Parliament Buildings more than the movie as reflected in her diary:

> A trip to Ottawa for Carol Ann and I. We drove to the capital (not to see Brian M) but to visit the parliament buildings and the Peace tower. It was all so interesting. I was very impressed with the library — it's worth seeing — just beautiful. Also, we had dinner the first night at a wonderful place right by the Rideau Canal. What beautiful scenery. Three great days — we saw lots of history. Thanks Carol Ann.

Not a word about her cancer, only positive memories and words of thanks. This was so like my mother.

Jamie and I took Mom to the Old Mill restaurant many times. It was always her favourite place to dine and we loved taking her there. In the middle of our radiation treatments Mom called me one Friday evening to ask a favour. "Let's get all dressed up on Sunday and go to the Old Mill for brunch. Let's pretend we have never had cancer. Promise me you won't even say the word once during brunch." I promised. Mom looked absolutely beautiful when I picked her up Sunday morning. She was wearing a bright suit with a matching scarf and a smile that would warm the world. She was feeling very ill that day and I knew it would not have been easy pulling herself together. Off we went with the promise to not utter the word "cancer" even once. A party of two cannot make a reservation at the Old Mill and as we parked the car we both observed a huge lineup to get in. I knew Mom could not stand in line but I had promised — I said nothing. We walked to the back of the lineup and about twenty seconds later Mom leaned over to me and whispered, "Here's what I want you to do. Go in there and tell someone I HAVE CANCER." So much for our pact! But it worked — we moved to the front of the line. There was a two-seater table that Mom and I had admired over the years and we wondered what one had to do to be seated at that table. Now we knew — a spot of cancer gets you the best seat in the house! The waiter immediately brought us each a complimentary glass of wine. (Mom didn't drink so I had two!) We laughed about this for the rest of Mom's life and it is one of my most cherished memories from our black humour files.

The next big excursion for Mom was to the military tattoo in Halifax. We had established a tradition of taking her home for the tattoo every year following her move to Ontario in 1984. Mom loved to see the different regiments marching on parade and the music of the bagpipes brought back fond memories. Connie flew in from Hawaii for the trip and we had managed to get front row seats for the show.

On June 30, before the tattoo began, Mom whispered to us that she had to go to the washroom. Barely back in her seat she had to get up again. Mom never complained about pain, so when she told us she was hurting we knew it was serious. We also knew she would not leave the tattoo unless it was absolutely necessary. Clearly something was happening.

We got her into a cab to go back to the hotel, then asked Mom if maybe we should go to the hospital instead. In her polite way she said, "Well, that's what I'd like to do, if you girls don't mind." After examining her, the doctor explained that she might need another radiation treatment to ease the pain in her lower back, where a large tumour was pressing on her spine. We spent most of the night in the emergency room and she rested the next day. She had one errand that had to be done. Lois would be turning fifty the next year and Mom wanted to buy her a MacAskill photograph. She allowed us to walk with her to the store but we waited outside while she made the selection herself. We would not see the actual photograph until Lois opened it for her birthday and she would not tell us which photo she had chosen. I had to fly back to Toronto the next day, but Connie and Mom visited in Halifax for a few more days. Mom knew this was her last trip home.

I had returned to work in June. The first day back at the office I felt different about being there. The daily problems we faced on the job were not life-threatening, and I was no longer as excited about climbing the corporate ladder. I had loved every second of my job, but knew it was time to move on. My open-door policy lent itself to many questions about my cancer and created the opportunity for my team to talk with me about their own cancer experiences. I felt I could give back to the cancer community in some way, but was unsure what that might be.

Lorraine warned me that I might be treated differently when I returned to work. She was concerned that I would assume everything was back to normal with my career and she wanted to prepare me for the possibility that everything would change. She had witnessed many similar scenarios throughout her nursing career and gave me an example of what I might face. Knowing my love of public speaking, Lorraine gave me an example that would apply to my situation: I might deliver the best speech of my life, and at the end someone in the audience would whisper, "She had cancer, you know," not having heard a word I said. Cancer would be the focus, not my fabulous speech.

One day I was out with my installation team and got caught in the rain. I went back to my office at day's end with my hair wet and two of my managers followed me to ask if I was feeling okay. Normally these guys would have made fun of me in my wet clothes with my work boots still on. A few minutes later, one of my peers came in to ask if I was okay and to suggest that maybe I had returned to work too quickly. He thought I looked thin. (Hello, I was thin *before* I had cancer!) I went into the ladies' washroom and someone else suggested I wasn't taking care of myself properly. Lorraine's words echoed in my mind.

By the end of my first week back on the job I knew my priorities had changed. I probably could convince everyone I was okay if I wanted to do that, but I decided to give my future some serious thought. More critical in my life was my mother's gradual decline in health. My sisters and I had realized that Mom should no longer be living alone. We decided to suggest to her that she move in with me. It was to be a bittersweet decision in many ways. I had imagined Mom and I living together in happier times.

Mary and "Her Girls"

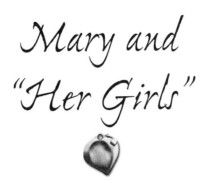

$\mathcal{I}$ took a deep breath as I unlocked the door to enter my home. I always needed a few minutes to gather my thoughts after a long day at the office, before greeting my mother on the other side of the door. Each day as I parked my car and rode the elevator to the ninth floor I tried to think positive thoughts. I wanted Mom to see me in an "up" mood as often as possible. My commitment to Bell was secondary to my commitment to her. Mom had moved in with me and I was determined to make her last months as pleasant as possible.

My sisters and I had spoken extensively about what would happen when Mom would no longer be able to cope on her own and should live with one of us. We knew that approaching Mom about this would be difficult; her independence was very important to her. Lorraine flew in for the weekend and we drove to Mom's apartment together. She did not meet us at the door, but quietly said, "Come in, girls," reminding me of the day she had been diagnosed. She was now very weak from the various medications she was taking and appeared very small in the chair facing us. Lorraine began the conversation by telling Mom we thought she should not be living alone. But before she could continue, Mom surprised us by saying, "I know I can't be alone any longer and I have to ask you girls to look after me." She didn't add "until the end," but it was implied. She had obviously been thinking about this on her own. Lorraine promised her we would always care for her and that we would never do anything against her wishes.

I invited Mom to move in with me. "I can't do that to you, Carol Ann," she said, starting to cry. "You have your own life." I tried to assure her that it would be easier for me because I wouldn't have to make the drive to Scarborough to visit with her. Lorraine and I could tell she needed some reassurance, so we suggested turning my master bedroom into a small apartment for her. She liked our idea and began to feel better about the plan. There were many things we could do to make it "our place." Knowing she was now feeling positive about it, we moved to specifics — what she could bring with her and when the move would take place. Lorraine suggested Mom should move before Labour Day, which was a month away. But Mom and I were very much alike once we made a decision, and the next morning I called Mom. "Let's do it now," I said. "Let me call a moving company and see if they can move you next weekend." Mom was already packing.

The week was a busy one as I juggled work with moving plans. I vacated the master bedroom area and left it empty for Mom's things. We would create her home exactly as she wanted it to be. Each day after work, Mom and I packed her things and made decisions about what would come with her and what would go to my cousins, Ed and Anna Taylor. They had always been very good to Mom and now were offering to store any of her furniture and personal possessions she couldn't take with her. She felt confident knowing her godchild would be caring for some of her things.

Throughout the entire process, Mom and I had only one argument. She had made the decision to not bring any of her dishes; she didn't want to invade my kitchen. Laughing, I reminded her that *nothing* happened in my kitchen and certainly there was ample room for all of her things. Mom's meals had always been very important to her. She dressed for dinner and used her good china. I wanted her to have her dishes and anything else that made her feel more at home, but she refused to budge on the issue. On moving day, the movers were separating the boxes — those to come with us and those to be taken to Ed and Anna's. When I saw the kitchen boxes clearly marked "storage" I quietly asked the movers to take them to my home instead. As we unpacked them later in the day we stood in the kitchen together and washed every dish before putting them away. Nothing was said about the disagreement and she used her good dishes every day.

I had asked Jamie to come down for the weekend and be with us on moving day. His sense of humour would lend a bit of levity to an otherwise sad day. He could always make his grandmother smile. Sure enough, Mom wrote what she was feeling in her diary, and although she didn't tell me directly, I knew she felt happy. Sadly this was to be her last entry:

Today I moved in with Carol Ann. I have a lovely small apartment and with all my own things it will feel like

home. As bad as things are for me I'll be happy and safe
here. I know the girls will always look after me till the end.

Living with my mother for the first time since I was a
teenager was difficult and extremely different, but we quickly
adjusted. Just prior to her moving in, Brian and I had discussed living together. This was a huge step for me and I felt
it was time to make a commitment. However, when it became
apparent Mom could not live by herself, Brian realized he had
to step back and allow me to do what I had to do. He moved
to an apartment across the street, but was with us constantly.
Brian loved Mom and she felt the same way. The three of us
spent a lot of time together, and Mom also recognized our
need for private time.

For the first month, Mom managed to follow a routine. She
was proud of herself — living in downtown Toronto, the big
city. She didn't stray too far from our apartment at Church and
Charles St., but always tried to accomplish something each day.
She would go to the bank one day, the post office the next, and
the drug store on the third day of the week. On Fridays we
would take ourselves out for dinner. Each morning Mom would
be getting up as I left for the gym at 6 a.m., and when I returned
an hour later she would be dressed and sitting at the table having
her breakfast. Suppertime for Mom was 5 p.m., so she had
always finished her meal when I came home from work. One
day I called to check on her late in the afternoon. I was in
Montreal and would be arriving home around 8 p.m. She was
having a very good day and offered to have supper prepared and
waiting for me. I said "Okay, but don't tell my sisters that you
are now forced to feed me." When I arrived home she sat with
me while I enjoyed my dinner. I jokingly asked for dessert, and

she replied, "I didn't have time to make it because I had to call your sisters to tell them you forced me to cook for you."

When Mom first moved in with me we had a celebratory dinner at a restaurant near my home. Boxes had been unpacked and Mom truly loved her little apartment. We had even sent a piece of my furniture out to be reupholstered to match Mom's couch. It was time to celebrate! We sat in the window seat at Giraffe restaurant and I was sipping from a glass of wine when Mom turned to me and said, "Carol Ann, I need to talk to you about my funeral. I would like to talk about it only once." I needed a second glass of wine as she spoke with such detail and calmness. "I don't want anything in Toronto, because your Bell friends will come and I don't really like your Bell friends," she said firmly. We laughed and I understood what she meant. She thought my life had always been too work-related, and if the people from Bell came to her funeral it would be because of me. She made it very clear that her funeral would be about her. I cried, but she did not. She was completely matter-of-fact. My feelings were in turmoil.

A month later Mom was beginning to feel weaker, and I was glad we had had the discussion. I noticed Mom wasn't even turning on the television or radio while I was gone during the day. She would just sit in a chair or lie in bed, and even sitting still seemed to take up all of her energy. When I asked if she found it lonely during the day she replied, "No, I'm just trying to cope." One day she added, "I'm sorry Carol Ann, I didn't think I'd live this long." It was heartbreaking to hear her say that, and I knew she felt like she was a burden to me. We talked briefly about what would happen near the end. The understanding Mom and I had was that when she felt the end was near, she would tell me it was time for Loarraine to come home.

Lois came again in October and Mom's spirits lifted. They took daily walks and managed to complete all of Mom's Christmas shopping. They strolled around Yorkville and stopped for tea so Mom could rest and observe the sights of Toronto. When they returned home Lois helped wrap all of the presents they had purchased, while Mom wrote a note to each of us — she was preparing early.

In late November, Mom's health was clearly deteriorating quickly, and I asked a friend to check in on her when I was at the office. For the most part, she was okay to stay by herself until I got home. But on December 1, I received a phone call at work telling me that Mom was very ill and was asking for me to come home. That morning I had left her sitting at the breakfast table and she had seemed in good spirits, although she was moving slowly. I drove back to the apartment in a panic, and when I arrived Mom was curled in a fetal position on her bed. I was startled by the change in just a few hours.

"Oh my God Mom, what has happened?" I asked.

"I'm afraid it's time for Lorraine to come home," she said in a whisper.

My heart was racing so fast I could hardly breathe. She was giving me the signal and it terrified me to hear the words. I said I would call Lorraine right away, but first Mom wanted a glass of water and a popsicle. I was crying and very anxious as I went to call my sister — I knew what to do but I couldn't make my hand pick up the phone. I stood in the solarium looking outside at the bright sunny day but not really seeing anything. I barely recall picking up the phone to ask Lorraine to come home. I know I sounded very troubled because only minutes later Lorraine's husband, Tom, called me back. He reminded me that the flight from Calgary would be four hours, but that Lorraine was booked on the next flight; I think he was actually calling to help me calm down. I was afraid to leave Mom for a second so I told Tom I would not be able to pick Lorraine up at the airport. As I hung up the phone I considered calling an ambulance to take Mom to the hospital, unsure if I could cope. The promise we made to her months earlier stopped me — I knew she wanted to be with her family.

The popsicle had melted and there was a large purple stain on the sheets when I re-entered Mom's room. I stared at it for a moment before telling Mom that I had called Lorraine. She looked at me and said, "Oh Lorraine, I am so glad you're here." I explained I wasn't Lorraine, but that she was coming and would be with us by the end of the day. Mom seemed to relax when she heard this, and her eyes focused on mine. She told me she wanted me to call her brother and sister in Hamilton and another sister in New Brunswick. She wanted them to know how bad it was — it was almost as if she had prepared a mental list of things that must be done. As I held her hand, she reminded me she did not want Jamie to see her this way and wanted to wait until she felt better for his visit. Mom was always telling me that Jamie's last memories of his grandmother should be positive ones.

I left Mom's room to call Connie and Lois. We had to discuss the need to change their existing plans to come for Christmas, which might have been too late. The plan had been for them to fly in on December 22 to celebrate Mom's birthday, Christmas, and Lois's upcoming fiftieth birthday together. Lois was unable to have time off work so would come as planned on December 22. Connie would arrive within twenty-four hours. Lorraine arrived a few hours later and took charge as she always did. I will never understand how Lorraine was able to be both daughter and nurse to Mom, but I will be forever grateful to her for it. When Lorraine was in the house I worried less. The next day Mom was feeling better, and was so happy to see Connie. She showed off "her place" and joked that she now lived downtown and no longer had to take the subway. This was a family joke, as Mom had never taken the subway!

Lorraine, Connie, and I decided we should make Christmas come early. We decorated our Christmas tree, hoping that Mom would soon feel well enough to come out of the bedroom and visit with us around it. Additionally, Lorraine told us about a jewelry tree she had seen in a magazine and wanted to create for us. She said, "Carol Ann, this tree will be classy and uptown — just like you." We decorated the tree with every single piece of jewelry we owned. If we needed earrings we borrowed them from the tree, but we understood that we had to return them by the end of the day.

We do have many happy memories. Each evening we would sit down for a nice dinner (my sisters are all good cooks) and we would share a bottle of wine. I had purchased my "Christmas wine stash" early, and we replaced it more than once. We traded memories from our past and laughed often. We could see Mom from the dining room so we were always able to keep a close eye on her. Many times two of us would encourage the third to get out of the house and go for a walk. But we could never leave the house for long. We wanted to be there for Mom, and for each other.

I worked very little during those final weeks and "the guys" were good to me. It was difficult to worry about work-related issues that seemed so trivial. I saw no need to get angry when we missed a key indicator or, God forbid, one of my guys had

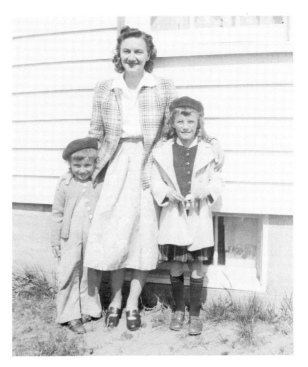

Me with Mom and Lois (note the tomboy look!)

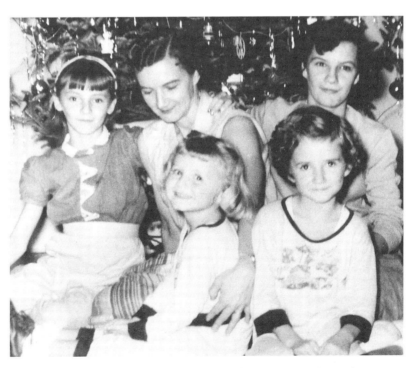

Christmas was always a special time for Mom and her girls.
From left, me, Mom, Connie, Lorraine, and Lois.

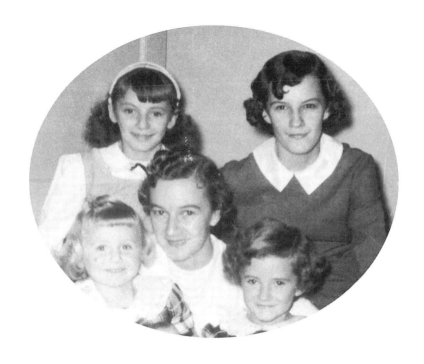

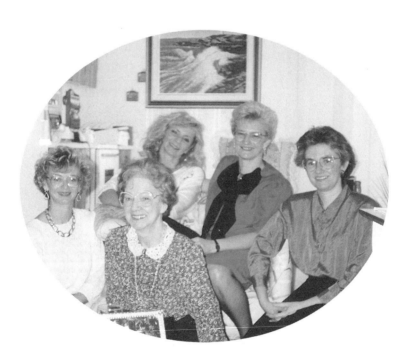

Mom and "her girls."

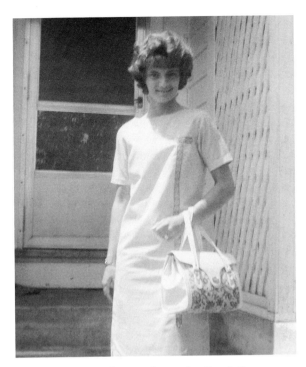

June 1964, leaving home for North Bay.

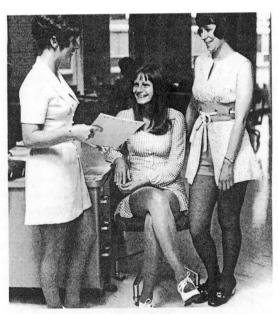

North Bay's Sally McLaren, order writer; Carol Ann Scott, service representative and Diane Bedard, service representative are in the office, but they've found a rather attractive way to beat the summer heat — it's called hot pants.

This appeared in the Bell newsletter in 1968. Not a great career photo op!

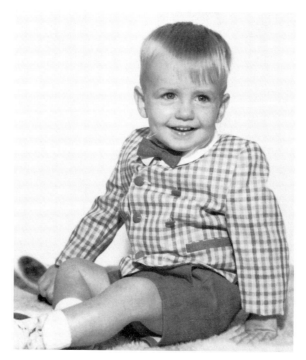

"The Boy," 1971

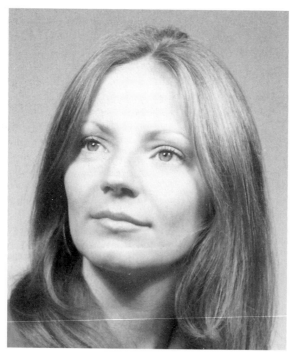

Juggling many responsibilities in Kingston, Ontario, 1973

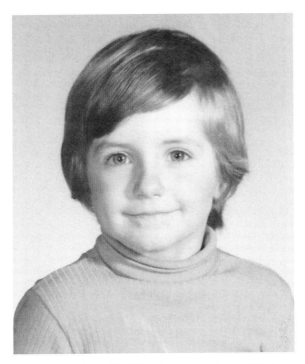

James in his official kindergarten photo, 1974

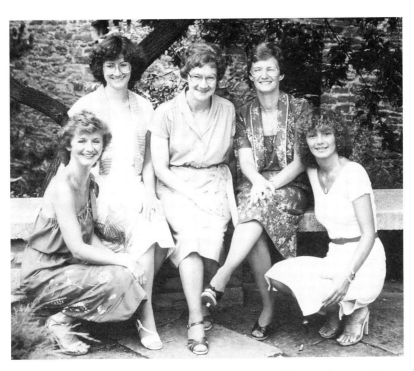

Celebrating Lorraine's marriage to Dr. Tom at the Old Mill, 1980 (he must have taken the picture!) From left to right: Connie, Lorraine, Mom, Lois, me

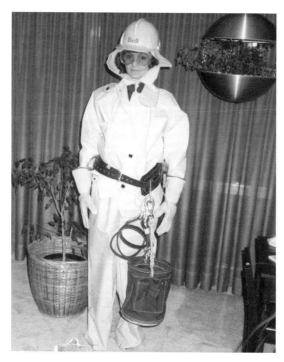

All dressed up and ready to move from the business office to Installation and Repair

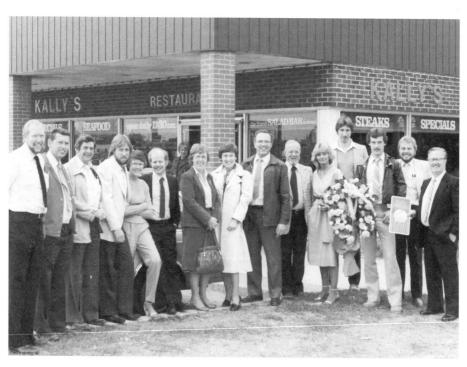

Saying good-bye to my Installation and Repair team, 1982

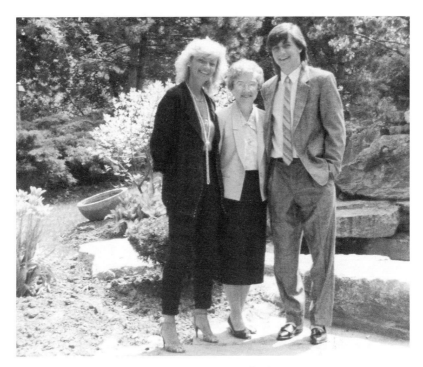

With Mom and James on Mother's Day, 1987

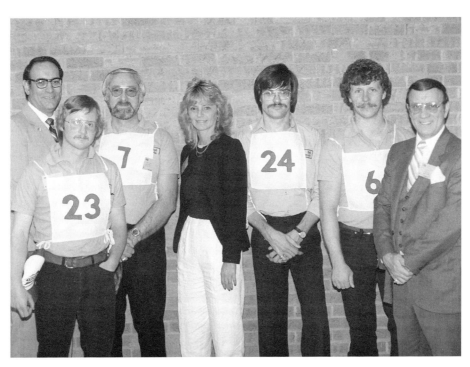

1984. My guys won at the Bell fork-lift competition

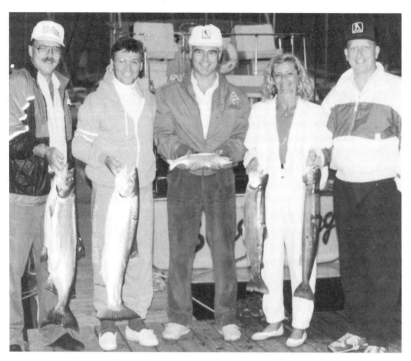

"Fishy business" with my boss, Mike Roach, and the Tele-direct boys

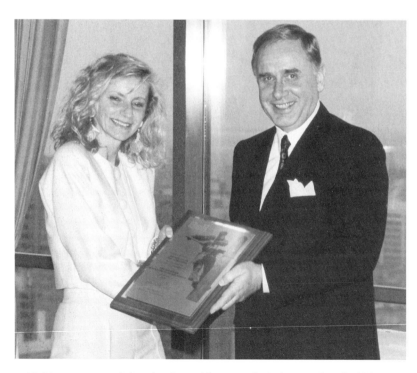

Murray Makin was a tough but fair boss (if you exclude his need to hold his meetings at the National Club, where women had to enter through the basement)

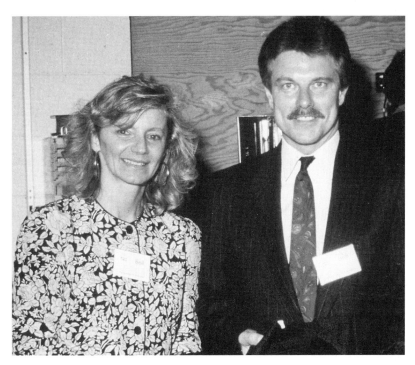

1989. I replaced Terry Mosey as VP Ontario South.
Terry later became President of Bell Ontario

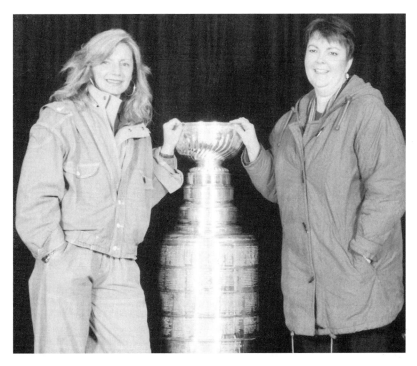

My secretary, Barb, and I with our "date," Stanley,
at one of the many Presidents' hockey tournaments we enjoyed together

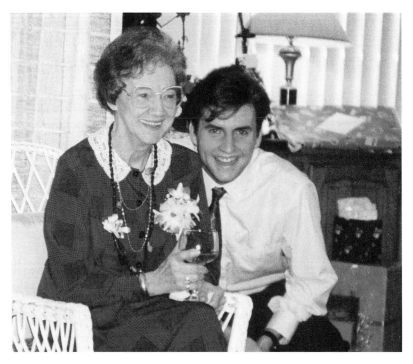

My Mom and James at her 75th birthday party in 1990.
My sisters and I have many wonderful memories of that magical evening

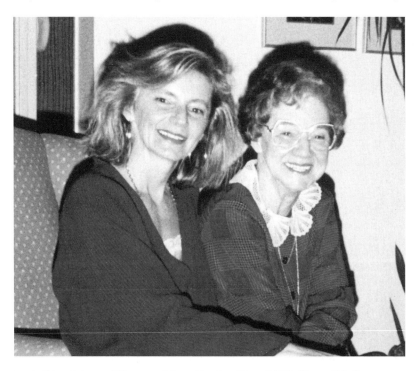

James took this picture of Mom and I on Boxing Day, 1990. Mom didn't approve of me
wearing "tights" and wanted James to zoom in so they wouldn't appear in the photo,
hence her big smile. I later used this photo in the Comfort Heart brochure

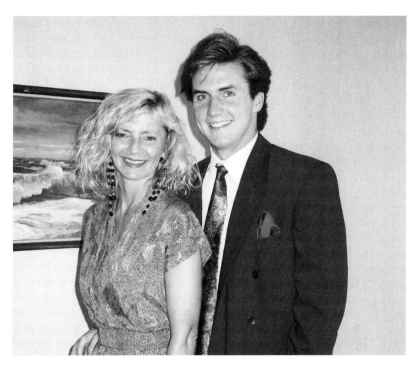

James and I in 1991

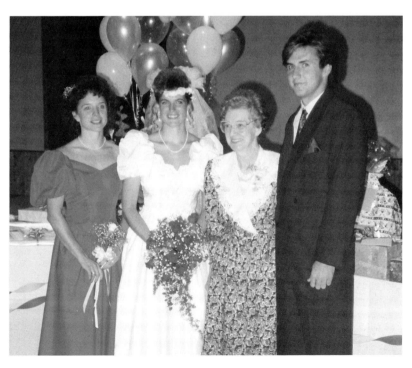

Mom with her three beautiful grandchildren at my niece Dawn Marie's wedding

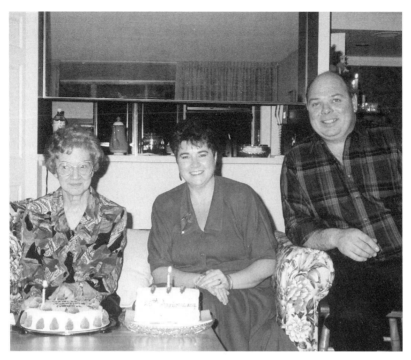

Celebrating Mom's birthday and my dear friends Donna and Randy's 25th anniversary

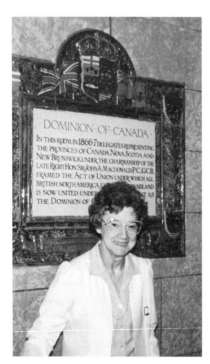

May 1992. Mom's last visit
to the Parliament Buildings in
Ottawa, Ontario

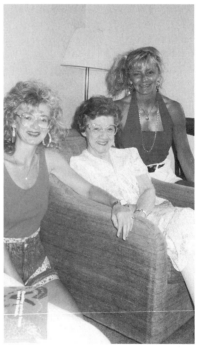

With Connie and Mom in July
1992, on Mom's last trip "home"
to attend the tattoo in Halifax

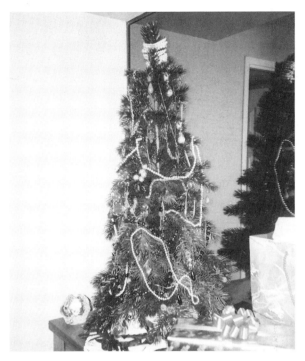

The jewelry tree that sat just outside of Mom's room

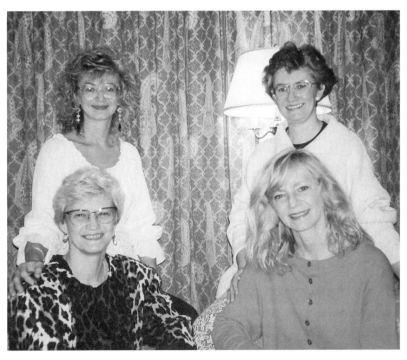

Taken just days after Mom passed away, you can see the pain behind
the smiles as we tried to pull together for Christmas

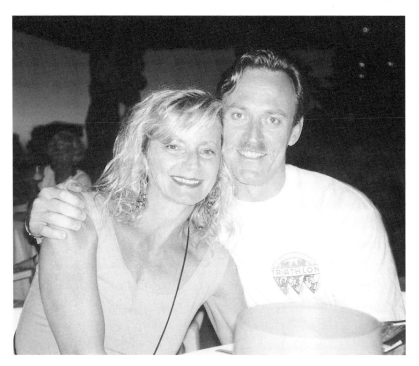

Brian and I share a bond that will last forever

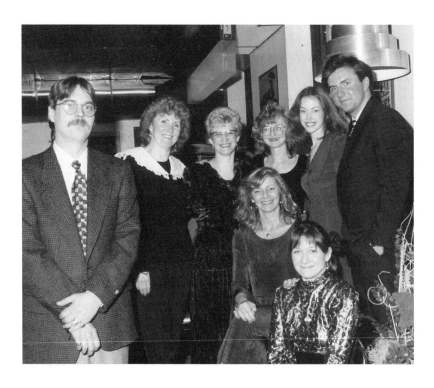

My retirement with my cousin Gary Curran, my close friend Phyllis Pedicelli, Lois, Connie, Tracey, James, and Gary's wife Lanis, seated

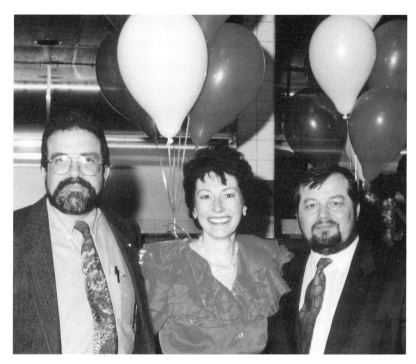

JC, Judy, and Sam, enjoying my retirement party

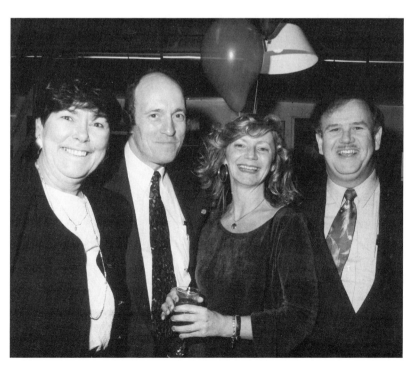

Celebrating my retirement with part of my team: Diane, Jack, and Bob

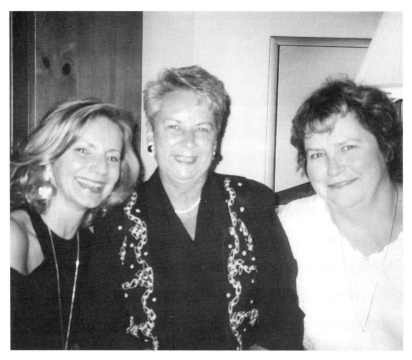

Carolyn Passmore and Kathy Service are
North Bay influences who became — and remain — good friends

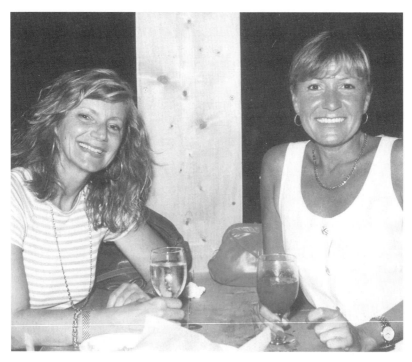

Teri McDowell and I attended the opening of Wayne Gretzky's patio restaurant and
wondered why Wayne and friends had been glued to a television in the corner.
We later learned they had been watching the O.J. Simpson Bronco chase

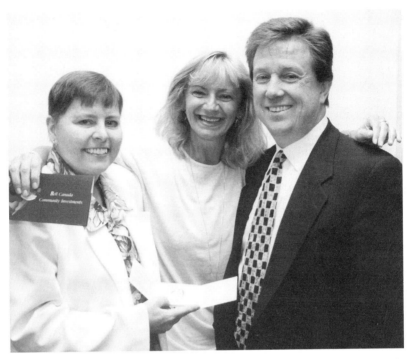

With Cathy Connelly and John McLennon (then President of Bell Canada) in 1996 as we launched the Comfort Heart Initiative

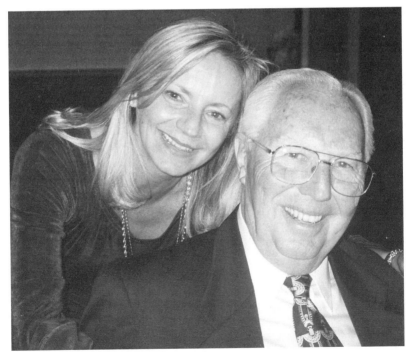

When Bell closed the North Bay office in 1997, I had the chance to, once again, thank Martin Kennelly for hiring me and mentoring me throughout my career

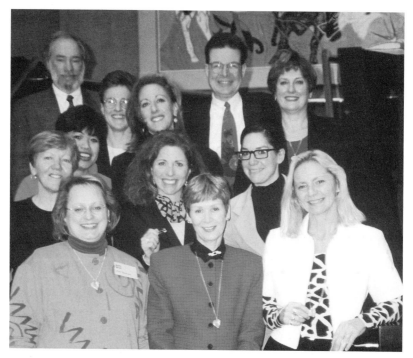

The Calgary Comfort Heart team, led by Hazel Gillespie, made a huge difference

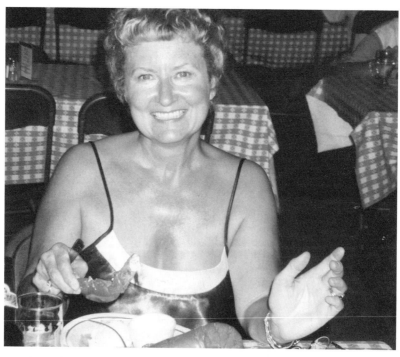

Cancer took my friend Trudy's life, but her smile lives on with all of us who loved her.
She enjoyed this lobster dinner while visiting with me in Nova Scotia

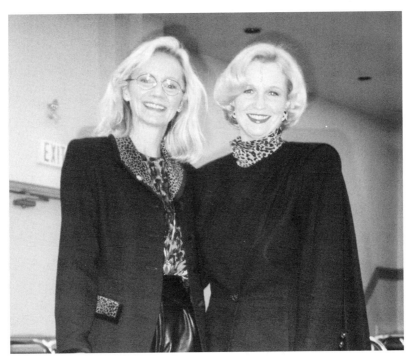

Ruth Foster is my greatest Bell supporter
(we are, what I call, the "Leather and Lace" team)

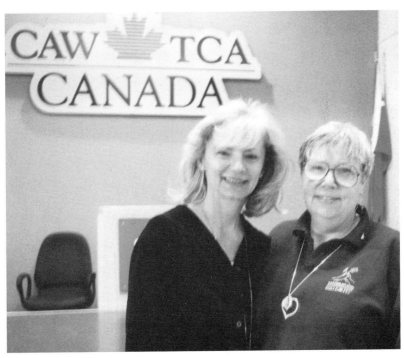

Marilynne Lesperance is the heart of the C.A.W.

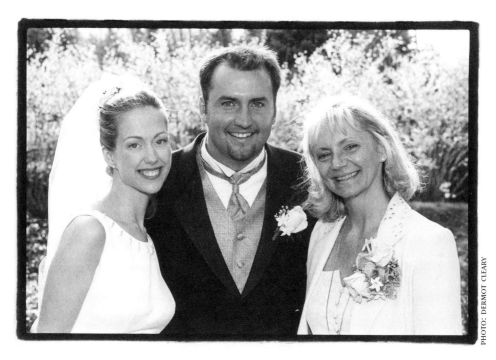

With Tracey and James on their wedding day

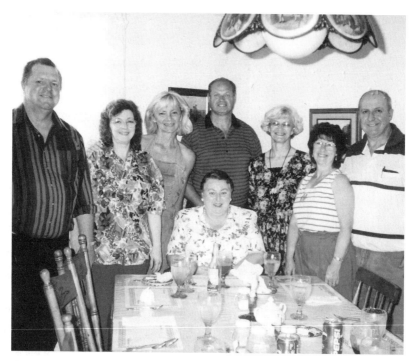

Family and friends celebrating with my cousin, Anna, on her 57th birthday at Café Chez Christophe. Ed and Anna represent, for me, the last of Mom's Acadian roots. Mom loved them both very much and was a very proud godmother to her niece, Anna.

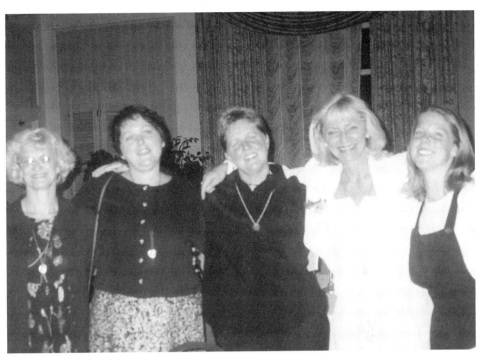

Lois and I with the OceanArt team: Linda Power, May Ocean, and May's daughter, Erin

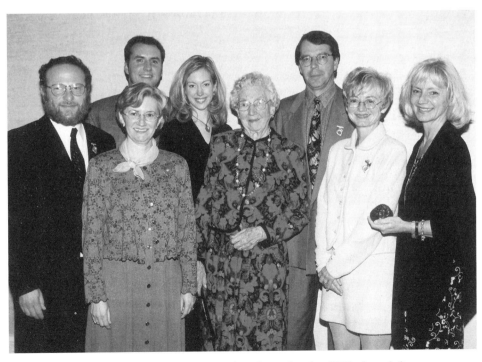

Receiving the Terry Fox award with my family, 1998, from left:
Lorraine's husband Tom, Lorraine, James, Tracey, Lucy Dea
(Connie's mother-in-law), Connie's husband John Dea, and Connie

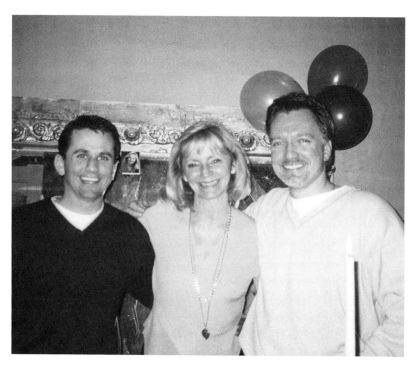

Celebrating with Francis and David.
I am one of the older women in their lives

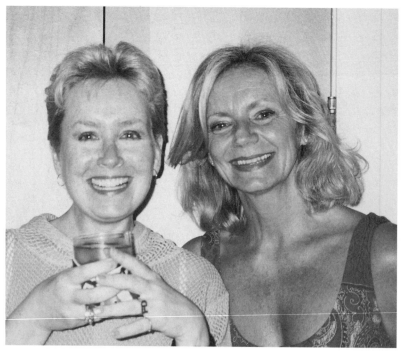

Faith at 50! We had a huge party for my good friend Faith in my small Toronto loft.
Her family and friends came from Florida and Chicago to surprise her.
Her father still talks about the party, so Teddy, this one's for you

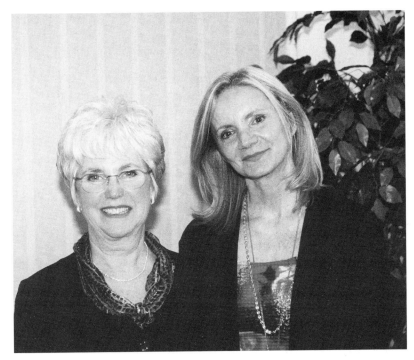

Carol Bond's annual "In the Pink
—Fun and Fashion Show" is much more than a fashion show

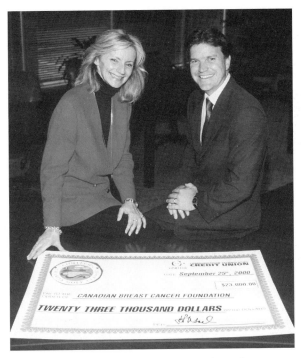

With John Mach, President of Comtech Credit Union.
They have purchased over 10,000 hearts to date and
have also raised $23,000 at a golf tournament

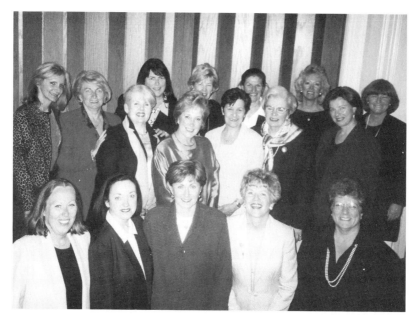

An "Order of the Heart" evening where I was toasted and roasted by the "Bell Babes"

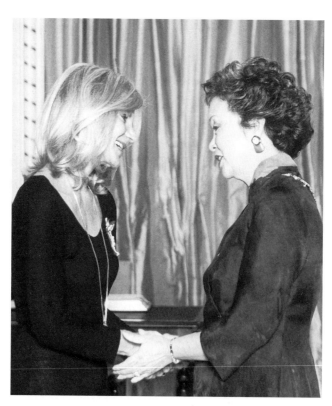

Receiving the Order of Canada from Her Excellency
The Right Honourable Adrienne Clarkson in May 2001

a motor vehicle accident. At the same time, a seemingly indifferent attitude doesn't necessarily let you keep your VP job for long. It was very close to Christmas and one evening we had a late meeting and decided to all go to dinner together. While the guys had a pre-dinner drink I hurried home to check on Mom and touch base with Connie and Lorraine. It was difficult to leave my emotions behind when I rejoined the guys, but they were waiting for me. It was a warm moment for me as they each found a way to let me know they understood what I was going through and that they cared. Over dinner, I told them I didn't think Mom would live to see Christmas.

Although Mom was very ill and often didn't feel like talking to anyone, she loved having her daughters with her. We would joke and tease each other so much that Mom told us we were acting like we did when we were kids again; she always made sure to include Lois in her discussions and encouraged us to call Lois often so she would not feel left out. I think as her first-born, Lois had a very special place in Mom's heart.

One day she took my hand while I was sitting with her, and out of the blue said, "I never did thank you for making me bring my dishes with me when I moved into your home, Carol Ann." She was still finding ways to give thanks and make others feel better, even when she was dying. I walked out of the bedroom after that comment and broke down in the living room. I could barely tell Connie and Lorraine what had upset me.

Mom had not spoken with Dad for many years. She asked me if I had been in touch with Dad and if he knew how sick she was. I had kept in touch and had visited with him briefly over the years, and he was aware that cancer had invaded our family. I asked Mom if she would like to speak with Dad and she said yes. They spoke a couple of times. She never told me what they talked about, but when Mom hung up the phone, tears were streaming down her face.

My sisters and I had developed a nightly routine to ensure someone was always close to Mom's bedroom; one of us would sleep on a mattress on the floor near her door. On December 20, it was Connie's turn to sleep on the floor, and we kissed Mom goodnight and went to bed. I realized I had left my glasses in Mom's bedroom and went to retrieve them. As soon as I saw her I knew death was near, and I quickly called out. We sat with Mom, holding her hands and telling her how much we loved her over and over. Her death was peaceful and she knew we were with her until the end — just as she had asked.

We then had to call Dr. Frank Ferris — the doctor from the palliative care team. Everything became a blur as we followed the procedures we had been given months earlier when we first began preparations to allow Mom to die at home. The hardest part was watching the men from the funeral home bring in a trolley with the body bag. Connie and I wanted to be with Mom and we even followed the body to the waiting hearse. We then called Jamie and he came home immediately.

The next few days were busy as we made funeral arrangements and booked flights to Halifax. Mom had told me she wanted to be cremated and have her funeral celebrated in Nova Scotia. She wanted Monsignor Terriault, who had been her parish priest in Annapolis Royal, to conduct the mass. She felt that he was the one who saved her life when Dad left. But first, we had to deal with Christmas.

It was almost impossible to celebrate Christmas that year, but we went through the motions because we knew it was what Mom wanted. Mom's Christmas presents for us were under the tree. We thought back to October when Lois helped Mom complete her shopping. Christmas had always been so important to Mom, and now it would be up to us. She had bought me a wonderful pair of silver earrings that year, knowing my love of jewelry. She bought Jamie a sweatshirt and he kept it in the box with the tag for over a year, not wanting to touch it. The MacAskill photograph that Mom had purchased in Halifax for Lois to open in celebration of her fiftieth birthday sat under the tree, and through our tears, Connie and I explained to Lois how important that purchase had been to Mom. She had selected the beautiful 1941 photo of the church in Grand Pré, Nova Scotia.

The next day was Christmas, and it was so difficult to do anything. Certainly there was nothing for us to celebrate. I was very weepy and had turned on the television for distraction. *The Prince of Tides* was airing, and it made me remember the previous Christmas when I had taken Mom to see it with Jamie.

Tom insisted that on Boxing Day he would treat us to dinner at the Sutton Place Hotel; all we had to do was dress up and arrive. Tom took our picture before dinner. It's hard to miss the sadness in all of our faces in the photograph, but it's one I cherish to this day. Tom gave us more than a gift of dinner that day.

Connie and I would sometimes wander into the room that had been Mom's bedroom to sit and think. Connie liked to sit in Mom's rocking chair to see if she could connect with her on a spiritual level. I would lie on her bed and think about the good times Mom had in that room, but it only made me miss her more.

We travelled to Halifax for the funeral, with Lois and Connie going a day earlier to make most of the arrangements.

Monsignor Terriault was now retired, but was happy to honour Mom's wish to have him celebrate her final mass. Many of her friends and family came — even some of the Cole women attended the funeral. I called Dad, but he didn't come. He had had a heart attack a few months earlier, and felt he wasn't well enough to attend. At the time I was furious that he wouldn't pay his respects to Mom, but in retrospect, the people who were at the funeral probably wouldn't have welcomed him there. The mass was everything Mom had asked for, and although our hearts were breaking, we knew Mom was now at peace. There is a saying that goes, "No matter how much other love you have in your life, when your mother dies, your world is cut out from under you." Lois, Lorraine, Connie, and I now knew that to be true.

I asked Ed and Anna to do me a favour while I was in Halifax. I couldn't imagine returning to my condo after the funeral and was anxious that some major pieces of furniture be removed before I came home. I thought if the condo looked even slightly different I could move forward. Nothing could have prepared me for the empty feeling as I unlocked the door. My home was everything to me, especially when you consider how fast-paced my life was with work. I thought of my condo as my sanctuary, but with Mom gone it just seemed empty. My heart ached one day when the settee Mom and I had sent out a few months earlier to have re-upholstered to match the décor in her room was delivered. Without my sisters to fill the void in the rooms I couldn't bear to be there. I knew it was time to move.

Perhaps it was time to start over.

Holders of
the Heart

"Early retirement" is something one thinks about and considers but never speaks of openly. A career could easily stall if you said, "Thanks for the promotion boss, and by the way, did I mention I will be retiring as soon as I qualify for a package?"

I had been given the opportunity to change jobs at the VP level. It was time to say goodbye to my Installation and Repair team. The position of VP Logistics offered the perfect job to truly test whether or not I wanted to continue my corporate climb. I worked with an entirely new team once again and enjoyed yet another learning experience. I loved the job and my new team, but months into the new job I knew it was time to move on. Connie moved home from Hawaii and I encouraged her to live with me until she found just the right job and a place of her own. After all, I had my job at Bell, a six-figure salary, a huge condo, and was thrilled with the idea of sharing it all with her. At that stage, moving on for me didn't include retiring.

In mid-November 1993, one of my managers and I were driving to a meeting. John drove while I studied the latest retirement package just released to the executive team for review. The "magic" number for qualification was seventy-five — age plus service had to add to seventy-five years or more. On average the magic number had been eighty-five or eighty in previous retirement packages. I quickly (and quietly) did the math: age (forty-seven years and nine months) + service (twenty-seven years and three months) = seventy-five years exactly. I qualified!

I immediately made an appointment to speak with my boss, Diane Chabot. I filled out the forms and anxiously sat across from Diane in her luxurious office on 10 South, unsure of how she would react. Initially Diane was shocked — *totally* shocked. She quietly asked if my cancer had returned, because she couldn't imagine why I would walk away from an executive position at forty-seven years of age. As I explained my rationale, she shared with me that she had met others who had beaten a potentially life-threatening disease and changed their lives shortly after. She reviewed my package, made suggestions regarding my entitlement, and agreed to review my request with the president. As I left her office she reminded me that, once announced, many would assume I was ill again. I would need to be sure that I was prepared for that reaction.

I met with a financial advisor, who felt if I could resist purchasing $2,500 suits at Chez Catherine in Montreal or leather suits from Harry Rosen in Toronto I would be able to retire and live comfortably on my pension. My years of paying down mortgages, not living on credit, and saving my Bell shares had paid off. My family was thrilled with my decision, although it gave Connie lots of ammunition — having just convinced her to move in with me, I would now be giving up the big salary and was already talking about downsizing my condo. So much for helping my little sister!

My last day on the job was pure magic. Everyone who had been important to me during my career found his or her way to my office. Gwen Guillet, who truly was a budget "expert" and had saved my hide many times, sent the most beautiful bouquet of twenty-eight pink roses — one for each year I had spent at Bell. All of the executive assistants on 10 South came, as a team, to my office to thank me for being so respectful of them, and installers from my previous jobs came in — work boots and all — to shake my hand. I couldn't empty my computer's inbox fast enough to keep up with the good wishes. I asked Connie to meet me at day's end just in case I was feeling emotional when it was time to leave. We walked out together and continued the celebration late into the evening. Clearly, my decision had been the right one.

At my retirement party in February 1994, one of the most precious gifts I received was a small book. "Fax it to me" was put together by my admin services team and contained a copy of all the e-mails and faxes I had received when my retirement was announced, and all those I had tried to keep up with on my last day. There were hundreds of notes nicely packaged for me to read again and again over the years. The party was everything I could have asked for. Teri McDowell put her expertise as an event planner to work and everything was perfect. Jamie and Tracey were picked up by limo in Barrie while another limo came to my home. Lois and Connie were with me, Phyllis came from Montreal, and Gary Curran came from

Thunder Bay with his wife Lanis. Gary is one of my three cousins with whom I had lived in North Bay with my Aunt Edith. There were many presentations and speeches. Perhaps the proudest moment of the evening for me was when Jamie stepped up to the podium. He made everyone laugh and cry. After all, he had the "inside scoop" on living with me and he took advantage of the moment. He reduced me to tears when he thanked me for driving him to Collingwood on sixteen consecutive weekends when he was eleven years old and wanted to become a world champion ski racer. Charlie Labarge was the master of ceremonies for the evening. Charlie had "taken a chance on me" and given me that first job in the Metro Machine, and he was still supporting me at my retirement party. When all the speeches were finished, everyone danced the night away.

First on my retirement list of things to do was sell my condo. Since Mom's death I had not been able to enjoy my home. My plan had always been to retire and move home to Nova Scotia but now I had difficulty doing that. My promise to my mother many years earlier had been that when she was eighty and I was fifty, I would retire and we would both return to Halifax. I didn't feel that I deserved to move to Halifax (at least not yet) so I sold my condo and moved to the Harbourfront in downtown Toronto. It was a beautiful place, but not truly my home. That would come later.

I had four goals when I retired:

1. Move (done!)
2. Find a way to give back to the cancer community through volunteer work
3. Launch my own professional speaking business

4. **Write a book about my career (I even had the title picked out — *10 South*)**

My relationship with Brian ended and we worked hard at remaining friends. It was a difficult breakup for both of us; Brian had been there for Mom and I through our cancer experiences and I knew I would always love him for that. He has a soft side that most men could learn from. For various reasons though, we were not on the same page.

Just after retiring I decided to visit my father. I had checked on him over the years, but never really visited with him. My Father's Day gift to both of us would be time together. I had planned to stay for a week, but the visit lasted only three days. He was still the same person I had remembered, absorbed with his own beliefs and unable to even talk to me about earlier years. Instead of dwelling on everything negative, I decided to leave and spend the rest of the time catching up with old friends. I visited with Mom at her gravesite and talked with her about my visit with Dad; sadly, my visit with Mom was more rewarding. I reconnected with my old high school sweetheart, Jerry Adams, and we shared years of stories. We spent a wonderful day together and en route back to the city we stopped at a little store called OceanArt Pewter. I wanted to pick up a few gifts for family and friends. I bought a gift for my son and each of my sisters and stood in line to pay. A little wicker basket filled with pewter hearts caught my eye. The hearts were called "Worry Hearts" and the insert card said, "Worry night, worry day, wish all your worries away." There was a thumb imprint on the heart and I stood rubbing it and thinking how soothing it felt. I bought a few of them quickly for my sisters and a few friends. But back in the car I couldn't stop thinking about the hearts and the simple message they conveyed. By late afternoon I was convinced those Worry Hearts would be perfect gifts for all of the people I worked with who had cancer and for some of my friends at Bell. My mind was racing as I made a mental list of names of the people I thought would gain comfort from this gift. I made Jerry take me back to the store, and bought over twenty-five hearts to take home.

"Hold the heart in your hand and think positive thoughts — create positive energy when you are going for your treatment or are worried about your doctor's appointment." I would repeat this to everyone to whom I gave a Worry Heart. Initially I gave them to women who were battling cancer, until one day a young telephone operator called me to say her mother had been fired and she wanted to give her Worry Heart to her mom — but only if I would give her another one because she couldn't go to her chemotherapy appointment without it. That gave me the idea that people outside of the cancer arena might also benefit from having a Worry Heart. I had been giving the hearts out only to women I knew, and never considered they might help on a larger scale. One day I got a call from John, who had been one of the managers at Bell. He was a large husky guy, and when he called me I thought he was making fun of my gifts. "Listen, do you have any more of those little heart things you keep giving to some of the girls?" he asked. He couldn't even say Worry Hearts because he was so embarrassed. But then he became very quiet on the phone and said, "I need one, I have cancer." I was touched that he had called and sent him one right away. Friends told me he kept it in his pocket, and sometimes he would take it out and frantically rub it with his large hand. From then on my phone would ring often with calls from the other men who worked at Bell.

They would ask me for "one of those heart things," like I had given John. The idea was definitely catching on; I had given out 117 of those little hearts.

While I was discovering the power of the pewter hearts, I was spending time — too much time — with cancer patients, and it was making me very sad. I couldn't seem to say no to anyone. Many of the visits were bittersweet. I spent a great deal of time with Bev, a friend of a friend from Bell, who was dying of breast cancer. I had been to the movies with Bev and helped her buy a wig, and some days she just wanted to talk. She called early one Saturday morning to say she would really like to visit me in my home and wanted to come right over. Bev was a woman I had not known prior to her cancer diagnosis but now we found the one thing that connected us, and it was a strong connection. She came with her husband, who helped her walk off the elevator and into my condo. She had to lie down immediately and as we made her comfortable on the couch, she turned to me and said, "Now, you know what I would really like to do? I would love to share a glass of wine with you." Her husband looked horrified and reminded Bev she certainly was not permitted to drink. She turned to him and said, "Why not, is it going to kill me?" We laughed as we shared a glass of wine at 10:30 on a sunny Saturday morning. She died only days later.

The emotional stress of watching people die was taking its toll on me; it kept bringing back memories of my mother. It was chipping away at my heart and while I knew it was helpful to others, it was not always helpful to me personally. Giving back to the cancer community had to be easier on me emotionally than this, I thought — there had to be another way.

I shared my story of the Worry Hearts and the feedback

from over 100 people who were now "Holders of the Heart" with Jackie McKercher and Gaye Scott, my colleagues from Bell. Their reaction was, "Why are you giving them away? You could sell them and raise money for cancer research. You could make a difference." I immediately disagreed. My plan had never been to speak publicly about what I was doing with the Worry Hearts. This was between me and those to whom I chose to give a Worry Heart. However, I slept on their idea and the next day I called several of the "Holders of the Heart." I wondered what they would think of the idea. Their reaction was a very positive one. "We could be your best salespeople," said one, while another confided, "I'm glad I got mine when they were free!" Collectively they felt they could sell many hearts because they would be telling their own story. It would appeal to everyone in their world. My answering machine began to fill up with messages like "When do we start selling Worry Hearts?" "Have you done anything yet?" "Have you got it all figured out yet?" One survivor's message was the most encouraging when she said, "Hurry up, Carol Ann; I have sold nine already and have to deliver them soon. Get busy!"

Jerry Adams told me that May Ocean owned OceanArt Pewter, so I sent her a letter. I explained that I had battled cancer, I was a Maritimer, and hoped to move home one day (all Maritimers say that). I told her that I had been giving her Worry Heart to cancer patients and that I had an idea of how we could use them to raise money for cancer research. I then listed all the changes I wanted: I wanted them to change the name from Worry Heart to Comfort Heart, which seemed much more positive. My friend Bob Ward had suggested we put a hole in it so men could put it on their key chain and women could put it on a chain to wear around their neck. I also suggested the addition of a second smaller heart imposed on top of the heart. That change would allow me to explain that the two hearts were a symbol of survivors and supporters working together, heart to heart. I wanted the insert card altered to acknowledge my mother's courageous battle with breast cancer. As if all of that wasn't enough . . . I also asked them to give up their net proceeds.

I mailed the letter and a few weeks went by. I worried. And then I got the call.

Linda Power, OceanArt's vice president, called me to say May had given her my letter and had left the decision regarding their involvement to her. She loved the idea and was proud to tell me OceanArt Pewter would gladly work with me to launch this fund-raiser. Linda then confided that she, too, was a cancer survivor. She had already battled cancer twice — once as a teenager and again as a young mother with three young boys. OceanArt Pewter had been looking for a way to work with the cancer community when my letter arrived. It was a touching example of the connection that exists between cancer survivors.

Many details had to be worked out. We would sell the Comfort Hearts for $10 with over $6 going to cancer research. The cost of the manufacturing, shipping, handling, taxes, and any other expenses would have to be covered with the balance. My involvement would be totally volunteer — not a penny of the $10 would ever come to me. I wanted this to be a national fund-raiser and approached the Canadian Cancer Society (CCS), offering to give the money to them. They agreed to work with me.

My initial plan was to raise $500,000. I was confident I could raise it in only a few months by approaching the presidents of Canada's largest companies. After all, I had been a VP and had many connections — or so I thought. Bell liked my idea and agreed to purchase 3,000 Comfort Hearts, which they gave back to the cancer community. Their gesture was an excellent way for a company to show they have a heart — pun intended. John McLennan, who was Bell's president at the time, received thank-you notes from cancer survivors who had received their Comfort Heart as a gift from Bell. Cathy Connelly and I met with John to receive Bell's cheque for $30,000, and the internal Bell newspaper ran a feature article on the Comfort Heart Initiative. We were off and running.

That was the good news. Other presidents and CEOs that I contacted either didn't call me back or called to say, "Good luck, but we aren't interested." I soon realized it might take longer than a few months to reach my goal. I would need brochures so CCS could send my story out to their divisions in each province. Ruth Foster was the associate director of communications at Bell. I had not met Ruth during my career at Bell, but we were now talking regularly. My initial letter had landed on her desk and she was dealing with my additional request for 100,000 brochures. Ruth agreed to have the brochures designed and printed for me. (I think she mentioned something about not coming back again, but I knew she was kidding, so I pretended not to hear her.)

I rented a post office box near my condo at the Harbourfront and waited for orders to come in. I waited. And I waited. We had lots of little things to iron out, but I was certain someone would be ordering a Comfort Heart soon. Wouldn't they?

In February 1996 we launched the Comfort Heart Initiative officially. The Canadian Cancer Society distributed my brochures and they took 2,000 Comfort Hearts to sell in their offices across the country.

One day I received a call from David and Francis. David's mother was battling brain cancer and his partner Francis thought it would be helpful to them if I could talk with David. We spent a wonderful evening in their backyard laughing and crying together. They had been unaware of my own cancer history. A strong friendship grew from that first evening and they became the first to sell Comfort Hearts in a retail store. You can always find Comfort Hearts on display at Yes.Ter.Year Interior Accents in Toronto.

On a personal level I was emotionally ready to return "home" to Nova Scotia. I hadn't kept my promise to my mother, but each time I visited her gravesite I felt her giving me permission to come home. I sold my home once again and moved to beautiful South Park Street in Halifax. I arrived before my belongings and decided to sleep on the floor of my new condo. Early the next morning my neighbours, Mae and Cec, knocked on my door with breakfast and fresh flowers from their garden. I was what Maritimers call a "back from away" — there are many of us who leave Nova Scotia but seem to return. If you moved to Nova Scotia for the first time we would call you a "come from away." I quickly settled in, had the Comfort Heart mail re-routed to Halifax, and continued with my fund-raiser.

In December of that year, I did an interview with the *Toronto Star* and they ran a huge article on Friday, December 13. It is true what they say about the power of the media: that interview sold thousands of Comfort Hearts from coast to coast. I could hardly carry the mail home each day and I soon became friends with the post office team. Kate was my first contact in Halifax and I gave her a Comfort Heart to help her understand how important all of this mail was to me. I would spend the entire day mailing out hearts, and loving every second of it. I included a personal note with each Comfort Heart in response to the many letters that came with orders. I sometimes had to make two trips back to the post office each day because I couldn't carry all of the orders in one trip.

One of the first letters I received following the *Star* article was from an inmate in a penitentiary. He sent a list of names along with a very touching letter saying he had long ago given up thinking he could make a difference, but after reading the article he knew there was one thing he could do. He had his monthly cheque made payable to the Comfort Heart Initiative and asked me to send Comfort Hearts to as many people on his list as the cheque would cover. I mailed the hearts out and some of those who received them called me to inquire hesitantly, "How do you know John?"

In 1996 I received a letter from a Mary Cole. Imagine how I felt standing at the post office reading my mother's name on the return address. I felt my mother was connecting with me through her. Mary's letter read:

> I was just diagnosed with breast cancer on October 11, 1996, to my shock and surprise. I too have followed in my mother's footsteps. I was only thirteen years old when I went through this with my mom, twenty-eight years ago. I felt devastated and helpless. Fortunately my mom is still living at the age of seventy-two. I can't tell you how shocked Mom was when I told her I too had cancer. You and your mom will always be in my prayers, for you have touched my heart.
>
> Mary K. Cole

In 1997, we reached our goal of $500,000, and I was ecstatic. I gave out "tough sledding awards" to many of those who had helped me reach this goal — an OceanArt Pewter Christmas ornament in the shape of a tiny sled. I engraved "$500,000" on the back of each ornament and then stroked through that amount and wrote "$1,000,000," thus introducing them to our new objective. I was confident that we could raise much more than $500,000.

CCS sponsored two national speaking tours over the next two years. In the fall of 1997, I spent forty-seven consecutive days on the road. I could never be a rock star for many reasons, including the fact that I hate checking in and out of hotels. My schedule read like a coast-to-coast bus tour. I scuttled through noisy airports, endured endless flights, and appeared before wonderfully attentive audiences both large and small. People would line up to tell me their own experiences and to tell me what the Comfort Heart meant to them. One man shared through his tears that his wife had just died of cancer and he had bought a Comfort Heart to give to everyone in their family for Christmas. He wanted to thank them for helping him through a rough time, and would encourage everyone to purchase more. Patricia Rees gave Comfort Hearts on what would have been her friend Sarah's fiftieth birthday as a celebration of what her friend's life had been, and she continues this tradition each year. Volunteers in support programs gave and received hearts with pride. New champions proudly took up the cause. One elderly lady waited in line to share her feeling that, "This Comfort Heart helps break down barriers. It reminds everyone we are equal in this battle and it allows the sharing of the most intimate thoughts." Until she received her Comfort Heart, she had never spoken the word "breast" aloud (and she lowered her voice even then).

Under Hazel Gillespie's direction, companies and organizations in Calgary worked together to raise thousands of dollars through the sale of Comfort Hearts. Hazel is Petro-Canada's national community investment manager. Calgary's mayor, Al Duerr, declared November Comfort Heart month and I made several trips to their beautiful city that month to thank them for "having a heart." Competitive agendas were set aside as all media teams covered the story. Judy Birdsell, my sister Lorraine, and others started a tradition that grew and spread across the country: they held a wine and cheese party where the price of admission would be to purchase, or agree to sell, twenty-five Comfort Hearts. They too raised thousands of dollars.

The most difficult audience for me was always one filled with senior citizens. In each face I could see my wonderful mother. When I mentioned the price of a Comfort Heart, I could see them take their $10 from their purses and wallets, ready to make the purchase as soon as I finished talking. One gentleman forgot to wear his hearing aid and proudly told the others at the end of my presentation, "I didn't hear a damn word she said." At least no one fell asleep.

During this time I reached a personal landmark: I celebrated five years of being cancer-free. My oncologist had cautioned me there was nothing magical about the five-year mark for a breast cancer survivor, adding that it could come back at any time. "I wish you hadn't told me that," I said, "because for me it *is* a big deal." I knew doctors didn't encourage the five-year principle but for me this was a turning point, because I chose to make it one. I took myself on a cruise! The first time I shared with an audience that I was now five

years cancer-free it was the survivors who started clapping first
— they understood.

By July 2000, we had raised over $1,000,000 for cancer
research, selling these little hearts one at a time. Many companies and individuals partnered with me to make a difference:
the Bell Logistics department where I had retired became
Nexacor (and now Profac) and the employees raised over
$20,000. Comtech Credit Union made an initial purchase of
10,450 hearts with the promise to purchase more. Their cheque
for $104,500 was the largest single cheque I've received. They
held the first ever Comfort Heart golf tournament. Bell continues to purchase hearts annually (and whenever I ask). Each
year I contact Ruth and ask Bell to purchase at least another
1,000 hearts for me to give out on their behalf. The internal
Bell News often carries an update on my fund-raiser and that
always brings an immediate influx of new orders from my
former teammates. Bell prints the thank-you cards that I send
with each order and when my stock is low I simply reorder
by calling Ruth. They have been incredible. Jack Fitzgerald,
who had worked with me at Bell, has personally sold over
1,000 hearts, sometimes driving across the city to sell just one.
No order is too small for Jack to fill. We joke that he had a
"back-order" problem at Bell, but not so with Comfort Hearts.
He fills orders on demand.

Cathy Tyszko and I have become friends, even though we
have yet to meet. I have received at least a dozen letters, notes,
and cards from Cathy telling me who she is ordering the latest
Comfort Hearts for and what she has done with her latest
"stash." One card from Cathy said, "You have to colour outside the lines once in a while if you want to make your life
a masterpiece."

One day I was with Andrea Grimm at the CCS national offices. Andrea had become a true champion and we were reviewing the project to date. Dorothy Lamont, CEO of the National Cancer Institute, came looking for me with a grin on her face. She told me I was to be awarded the Terry Fox Citation of Honour for my work. I was surprised and thrilled to be hearing this from Dorothy. The note she sent me once the announcement was made is one of my most cherished possessions:

> Your dream and your dedication to that dream has captured the "hearts" and hopes of so many — it's wonderful! It was the highlight of my week to be able to tell you about your being awarded the Terry Fox citation. It's well deserved and I hope it provides opportunities to sell more hearts as well as doing its primary job . . . to honour one very special lady. Actually, let's make that two very special ladies — you and your mom.

I remember distinctly, as do many Canadians, when Terry Fox's run was halted in Thunder Bay, and we were all saddened that he had not reached his initial goal. To be granted this award, in the memory of a man I considered a hero in the fight against cancer, was a great honour. Even more inspiring was the fact that the award was also a special tribute to my mother, since everything I did with the Comfort Heart Initiative was in her memory. As I walked to the podium the night of the award presentation, I thought of her. I think she would have been proud of the Cole name as I accepted the award.

Aside from the Terry Fox award, the Jewish Women

International of Toronto named me their 1999 Woman of the Year and I was extremely honoured and humbled by their recognition of my work (to this day people think I'm Jewish because of it). The Canadian Auto Workers Women's Networking Committee gave me their CAW Eastern Women's Networking Region Award as Canadian Woman of the Year 1999.

When I was named to the *Maclean's* 13th Annual Honour Roll I was truly touched by the many cards and letters I received. The most touching letter came from a woman named Beulah. She called asking me to send Comfort Hearts immediately and she followed up with a long letter. She wrote to share with me that her daughter-in-law had died of breast cancer and that her son Randy had been having a very difficult time. Beulah's husband believed he was receiving messages from his daughter-in-law in his dreams and the message was always the same — "Tell Randy to wear the locket." They asked everyone, but no one knew of a locket. Beulah's letter went on to say,

> So, a couple of days later, Dad was going through the December 21st issue of *Maclean's* magazine when we flipped the page and there was Carol Ann Cole and her Comfort Heart. Dad nearly flipped and he said, "My God, there is the locket!" So I thank you for sending our lockets. I will let you know how Randy is doing down the road. My thoughts and prayers are with you and your sisters.

My initial plan had been to give five years of my life to the volunteer community, working non-stop with the Comfort Heart Initiative and then moving on. As I closed in on the

five-year mark, I knew I would move forward with other pro-
jects, but the Comfort Heart Initiative would never end. Over
160,000 people own a Comfort Heart today, but my work is
not done; there are still millions of people out there waiting
to purchase a Comfort Heart and to join my team that I affectionately call "Holders of the Heart."

Giving Back as a Volunteer

After moving home to Halifax, a friend from Montreal called out of the blue. We shared the bond of divorced women working in the corporate arena and often exchanged stories — both business and personal. Having read about the Comfort Heart Initiative in the paper, she called to say, "I just read about all the good stuff you are doing, but they don't pay you, do they? You're not earning a cent with this job, are you?" By her standards I was not getting "paid." The payment a volunteer receives, however, is far more rewarding than the almighty dollar and every volunteer understands that.

At a board meeting with a non-profit organization during my VP days we were introducing ourselves before the meeting began. I observed that those of us with a title used it when introducing ourselves, but volunteers said, "I am just a volunteer." I vowed at that time to find a way to convince volunteers that their jobs were more important than all the VP jobs combined. I would find a way to remove the word "just" from their vocabulary.

The work I've done with the Comfort Heart Initiative has been the most rewarding "job" I've ever had. We passed the first million-dollar mark and letters continue to arrive daily. Clearly this fund-raiser will live on and on. I absolutely love mailing out the hearts and I love hearing the stories that so many choose to share with me. The Initiative has certainly brought out the best in people. Many send money to cover the purchase of a Comfort Heart plus a donation to the Initiative.

A letter from Alaska was proof that our fight has no boundaries and that the connection between cancer survivors continues to be incredibly strong. It was written by a breast cancer survivor named Kathie who had received a heart from a friend of hers, another breast cancer survivor. She was asking if I could ship the hearts to her in Alaska: "I wanted to say 'hello' from your sister breast cancer survivors in the United States. Thank you for such a beautiful way for us to unite in our struggle against breast cancer." The order form that Kathie used was copied from the Canadian Cancer Society Web page. After reaching our revised goal of one million dollars, I needed to take exclusivity away from CCS and allow other organizations to participate, because I had received many calls during the first five years asking if others could work with me. Comfort Hearts will always be available through CCS, but I now have other partners as well.

The Breast Cancer Coalition of Rochester, New York has become my first partner outside of Canada. I am thrilled to be working with them. To date they have sold 3,900 Comfort Hearts and share with me some of the wonderful stories they hear regularly from survivors who purchase them.

In the fall of 2000 I partnered with the Atlantic Division of the Canadian Breast Cancer Foundation (CBCF) and we travelled throughout the four Atlantic provinces during Breast Cancer Awareness Month. For more than two weeks we "took to the road" and were often scheduled to appear in more than one city or town on the same day. I flew to Labrador West and the townspeople had a potluck dinner for me upon my arrival. The next morning a huge snowstorm swept through the town, and I feared no one would show up for our event. I should have realized that people from Labrador are comfortable with all types of weather (this was not a storm by their standards) and eighty-seven people showed up! The message I delivered was about breast health but given my reputation as "the Comfort Heart Lady" we sold hearts as well — exactly eighty-seven of them. Everyone in Labrador seemed to know who I was and total strangers would stop me on the street to shake my hand and thank me for coming to their town. Many people even showed up at the airport to see me off and thank me once again.

In Fredericton, New Brunswick, I participated in my first "Titz and Glitz" event. A group of local women had organized the evening to promote breast cancer awareness in a very innovative and unique way. The idea for Titz and Glitz was born in Halifax and has become an annual event there as well. Women come to the party decked out in bras they have decorated. I had pinned forty-five Comfort Hearts to a sports bra and when I got up on stage to talk, I whipped off my leather jacket for everyone to see. It was a fun event and the message of the evening was to celebrate life and have a good time, as well as to raise awareness.

And then there was my "accident" with the CBCF pink ribbon. You have undoubtedly seen many pink ribbons related to breast cancer, but trust me, you have never seen *this* pink ribbon. It is about ten feet tall and Deborah Grant, CBCF's executive director, insisted on taking it everywhere with us on the tour. We were rushing to pack up and leave Stellarton because we were due elsewhere and with the miserable weather we were anxious to get on the road. It was raining and the wind was blowing very hard. Deborah was carrying boxes and I offered to carry the pink ribbon to the car. Somehow, the wind caught the pink ribbon, my umbrella, and me, picked me up with the ribbon still firmly under my arm, carried me through the air, and then put me down rather gently about ten feet away, with the pink ribbon on top of me. As this was happening, three young men approached me and one said in a very confused tone, "Is anyone seeing what I'm seeing? This woman is *in the air*. Is she flying?" They picked me up from under the ribbon and helped me to the car where Deborah was still leaning into the car packing boxes. I remind her often that CBCF truly swept me off my feet!

The only reward a volunteer ever expects is a simple "thank you." When we finished the tour Deborah invited me to the office for a small celebration with her team. They gave me some wonderful gifts and I was truly overwhelmed by the "thank you" messages in cards from each of them. The most personal came from Hilary, who wrote:

> My heart aches more now, almost six years after the loss of my dad, than it did during his illness. I used to love telling his story/my story/our story about his death because I am so proud of him. Listening to you tell your

story over and over and over and over again brought my
dad's story to the front of my mind, as I am sure it does to
so many others. I have not told this for a while, but since
dissolving into tears (listening to you speak) and sobbing
like I haven't since his spirit left his body, I know how
important communication is and how powerful it can be.

Some of my most rewarding volunteer work is with the
Canadian Breast Cancer Research Initiative. CBCRI is a unique
Canadian partnership of the public, private, and non-profit sec-
tors committed to beating breast cancer. Whenever I do an
interview for CBCRI, the interviewer reminds me not to list
the seven partners, because they think it's "dull." But how can
the story of seven groups who park their egos at the door to
raise millions of dollars for breast cancer research be dull? With
that said, the seven partners are: the Avon Flame Foundation;
the Canadian Breast Cancer Foundation; the Canadian Breast
Cancer Network; the Canadian Cancer Society; the Canadian
Institutes of Health Research; Health Canada; and the National
Cancer Institute of Canada. I believe CBCRI is a unique partnership in North America — maybe in the world. It was created
in 1993 as a result of a groundswell of support from Canadian
women, activists, survivors, and women in Parliament
demanding focused attention on breast cancer. We are Canada's
primary funder of breast cancer research, and provide leader-
ship and expertise to reduce the incidence of breast cancer,
increase survival, and improve the lives of those affected by the
disease. I am proud to say that since CBCRI was formed in
1993 it has granted $71.5 million to 245 research projects cov-
ering the entire spectrum of breast cancer research, including
prevention, early detection, treatment, fundamental laboratory

investigations, quality of life, and health services. This is great news for families living with breast cancer. Each dollar spent on research brings us closer to beating this terrible disease.

As vice-chair of the management committee I am privileged to work with Dr. Kathleen Pritchard, our chairperson, and our outstanding volunteer team of top breast cancer experts and survivors from across the country. We meet four times annually (and as often as required via telephone) to develop the strategic research plans and to manage the research program. Together, we've come up with some pretty exciting programs to answer fascinating research questions. Can breast cancer be detected using hair samples? Can a newly identified gene be used to develop a treatment for breast cancer? With the best researchers in Canada working on these issues, we hope to find out the answers to these and many other baffling cancer questions. For me it is a "hands-on" opportunity to work with other survivors, as well as the best researchers in Canada. After all, one of these researchers may be the one to find the cure!

In 2001 we held our second Scientific Conference in Quebec City. At the Reasons for Hope conference we heard details of the newest developments in breast cancer research, talked with and learned from scientific experts, and shared a quiet moment with other members of the team.

I love volunteering each year at Carol Bond's In the Pink Fun and Fashion Show. This is her way of giving back and there is so much emotion in her fund-raiser. Carol owns her own business — New Women Prosthetics and Apparel. Having lost a breast to cancer over twenty-five years ago, she opens her home to survivors so they can see products available to them in private. Her fashion show is for women only (we don't even allow her husband Tom to attend the fashion show despite his work in preparation of the event). Carol's models are all her customers; they are survivors. The event showcases the survival and beauty of a woman who has lost a breast to cancer. From the first second Carol steps up to the podium we are on our feet. We cry with her and we laugh with her. We clap so much our hands hurt and when she says, "That's our fashion show ladies, thank you for coming again this year," we share a glass of wine with her. Each year when I plan ahead to determine the events I will give my time to, I always make sure I'm there for Carol!

Not all of my volunteer work is with the cancer community (believe it or not!). During my Bell days I had some fun and exciting times with the "A Team" — the Algonquin Council of the Telephone Pioneers. I loved working with the A Team. We held fund-raising events, helped the homeless, bought gifts for single women and their children when they couldn't afford them, and hosted the annual Christmas party for the Good Neighbours Club, which is a support system for homeless men.

I was president of the A Team when I became a VP at Bell and fund-raising suddenly became easier; no longer did we have to collect slightly used socks, because I could expense new ones. We had so many fun times together and even had the opportunity to sing the national anthem at a Toronto Blue Jays home game. Bonnie was in charge of looking after me on the field because I was very nervous — at one point she was actually holding me up. My first and probably last opportunity to be at centre field and Jamie was late getting to the game! After moving home to Halifax I missed a number of the Good Neighbours' Christmas parties, and when I finally did show up one of the men was quick to remind me that I had been missed. As I approached his table offering coffee, he said, "Hey Blondie, where have you been? You haven't even bothered with us for a very long time. Had better things to do, did ya?" Volunteering is a gift.

Colemind

When my son was very young I used to sing Harry Chapin's "Cat's in the Cradle" to him, a song about a father who always seems too busy to play with his son. Although Chapin wrote about a man's feelings, I still believe the 1974 hit could have been written about me and I have always substituted "Dad" for "Mom" in the song. In December 2000, James called to discuss Christmas plans, and he asked me, "Mom, tell me again what the words are in the 'Cat's in the Cradle' song — the part about you being retired?" I quickly recited the last verse for him, where the parent calls her son to see if they can get together, but the son doesn't have time.

James was asking me to recall the song because he was trying to tell me he had a ski contract in the Ottawa area on Boxing Day, meaning he would have to leave late on Christmas Day. In other words, I was invited for Christmas, but Christmas would end when his job dictated. After we talked, I realized the song really did ring true; James had become just like me.

That year James and Tracey were hosting their first Christmas in their new home in Barrie. They married in 1998 and I am fortunate to have a wonderful daughter in Tracey. She is an intelligent and beautiful young woman just beginning her own climb up the corporate ladder, and I am proud to mentor her on that journey. I consider her a friend. Tracey has heard me say often that James and I grew up together and she is totally supportive of our relationship. James and I seem to have something to talk about every day and find a way to connect either through e-mail, phone, or in person when I am in the Toronto area. He would tell you that he is a "Mama's boy and proud of it."

Christmas in our family has always been a huge event. Since my mom's death there have been years where we struggle to keep it special. It was such a wonderful time of the year with Mom directing all of us and bringing us all together without effort. With her gone it all seems to take considerable work. I think many families experience this with the death of their mother and I have found that acknowledging this difficulty helps.

On Christmas morning Tracey's parents arrived with her Baba and her brother Jamie. Shortly after, my sister Connie arrived with her husband John and the party continued. There is a tradition in Tracey's family that you guess what is in each gift prior to opening it. I failed miserably but am already practising for next year. Tracey and her brother Jamie have it all down to a very fine science. They not only guess what is in each gift from their parents, but they can tell you the colour and size. Not having my own mother there, I loved Baba most of all. She came into James and Tracey's home for the first time, looked around and said, "No drapes?" Only a grandmother can make a statement like that and get away with it.

We opened the pile of gifts and shared many memories of other holidays. James kept a running commentary about how his presents had changed since he married Tracey — instead of cool things he now only receives candles and potpourri. He was telling us this as he unwrapped a present from Lorraine and Tom. As he went on and on about the neat gifts Aunt Lorraine used to give him — a telescope one year, a tiny flashlight another year — he got the box opened. It was filled with candles. As we all laughed, James turned to his wife and said, "Tracey, this is all your fault."

Since Mom's death I had always shunned Mother's Day because it seemed to emphasize how much I missed her presence in my life. At Christmas, James finally talked to me about it, sharing with me that he felt sad he could not properly celebrate Mother's Day. Following Mom's death, he had never even sent me a card acknowledging the day, knowing how much it reminded me of losing Mom. But James felt it was time for me to "get over it" and move on with my life. He asked me if I would consider celebrating the upcoming Mother's Day at the Old Mill. He told me, "It was not just Grandmother's favourite place, but it's mine as well." I realized it was time to stop mourning and agreed to join him for lunch.

Five months later I found myself sitting at the Old Mill restaurant on a sunny Mother's Day sharing lunch with Connie, John, John's mother, Lucy Dea, James, and Tracey. James was worried that I would be upset seeing all the families with their mothers, but it allowed me to reminisce about all the other happier times we had celebrated at that restaurant. The lunch also gave me the perfect opportunity to give

James something that I had been keeping for a long time.

When James was born in 1969, I did not have very much money and so for Mother's Day I sent my mom a silver dollar commemorating the year her first grandson was born. I knew she treasured it and I saw it again years later when she moved in with me in the summer of 1992, as she had placed it in her bedside table. She told me that she wanted to give it back to James as something to remember her by — a gift not only from her but from myself, as a celebration of his birth. As her condition deteriorated, she didn't want James to see her that way, and fretted over when she would have a chance to give him the coin. To put her mind at ease I told her I would keep the coin for her, and when she was better we would both give it to James at the Old Mill. I tried to be light and joking with her, even though I knew that day would never come — she was already too ill. After Mom died I put the coin away, knowing that one day I would honour Mom's wish, even if she couldn't be there. This Mother's Day lunch provided me with the perfect opportunity.

I gave the coin to James after lunch as we were leaving the restaurant. I felt my mother smiling down on me as I put the coin in his hand, and our first return visit to the Old Mill felt right. Since lunch had been such a happy occasion, I told him I would explain the meaning behind the gift at a later time. I knew that I could not tell him in person because I would start crying, so I decided to send him an e-mail instead. His reply exemplified why I am so proud of this wonderful young man:

This might be one of the best stories you have ever told me. Happy Mother's Day. I thought of Grandmother today

as I always knew that you like to be with her at the gravesite on this day. The thought saddened me as I don't wish to know what it must be like to go through this day as you and your sisters do. I kept those thoughts to myself because I didn't want to upset you or Connie.

James is now a CSIA Level Four (Canadian Ski Instructors Alliance) and an Assistant Pro with the CPGA (Canadian Professional Golfing Association) so he has his winters and summers covered. He also returned to college to complete the education he first walked away from as a teenager when he wanted so badly to do nothing but ski. He does his "homework" on the very same antique desk that I purchased when I was first promoted to VP at Bell. I have passed it on to James and Tracey with the hope that it sees them through even more successes than I enjoyed while using it. I have also promised to pass my Mazda Miata on to James when he graduates. I must have made that promise in a weak moment!

Years ago, my decision to retire was made easier because I had a dream in which I received advice from my mother. At forty-seven years of age I knew I wanted to stay connected to the corporate world while giving much of my time and energy to the cancer community. In my dream Mom advised me to retire, work for myself, use my mind, and continue to do good things for the "Cole" name. When I got up the next morning I said to Connie, "I've made a decision. I am going to retire, start my own professional speaking business and call it 'Colemind.' I'll do some type of volunteer work too, but right now I have no idea what that will be." Connie jokingly remarked, "You made all those decisions during the night? Where were you?" I told her I had been with Mom, and she understood.

I registered Colemind just a few days after I retired but then put it in my "pending file" for five years so that I could give back to the community for that period of time. I continue to do many volunteer speaking engagements but also work with companies and businesses seeking speakers to motivate their team.

In many ways not much has changed. One of my most popular talks, "Glass Slippers and Glass Ceilings" relates to the struggles women faced at the time when I was starting my career, and are still facing today. The Famous Five Foundation in Calgary is involved with an event called "Rising Stars" and I had the pleasure of being their keynote speaker one year. They bring together 500 high school girls and it was so rewarding to hear their many questions and comments after my talk. A number of them even wanted to help me sell Comfort Hearts and stayed in touch to explore that possibility.

Being a professional speaker is not about the money you make (although to be honest, I have enjoyed that part of returning to the corporate arena). It is about having the privilege of speaking with an audience and helping them in some small way. When someone comes up to me after listening to my presentation and tells me how it has affected them I am truly honoured. Even more so if they tell me what they have learned will help them in their personal life.

I live my life at half past cancer. I have always been concerned when people have cancer and then say, "I want my life to be as it was before this happened." It's not that simple. I try to encourage them to understand that life will never be as it was before, but that's not necessarily a bad thing. Even though I no longer have cancer, I still devote half my time to giving back to the cancer community, while the other half of my life is outside the cancer world. Living my life at half past cancer allows me to hear about and perhaps understand the personal lives of friends living with cancer. When a friend apologizes for "bothering me with their cancer problems," I remind them that my volunteer work is very separate from being there for a friend confronted with this killer disease. As I write this book three very special friends come to mind:

Donna and Randy have been part of my life since I was sixteen years old. Several years ago Randy was diagnosed with malignant ocular melanoma — eye cancer. They enjoyed some good years after the original diagnosis, but it came back and has spread to his liver. Donna is Randy's friend, wife, lover, nurse, and doctor through this time and I am more proud of her today than ever before. We see each other when we can, and we e-mail daily. When Randy was first diagnosed he was told that his cancer was "one in a million." Donna and Randy are two in a million!

When I first met Pat I called her my "limo-lady" and now I call her my friend. She picked me up one day at the airport and has been driving me back and forth ever since. She listened to all of my half past cancer stories, I listened to her, and we formed a special bond. Pat has already been through more than any woman should have to endure. Life has dealt her many hardships and each time she has accepted her fate and bounced back from personal tragedy. One day when I called to book her for an early morning flight she asked if she could pick me up a bit earlier so we could talk — she had something to share. I knew without asking: cancer had knocked on her door. She had a cancerous tumour in her mouth and surgery would include hollowing out her cheek, removing all the muscle, part of her jaw, and her lymph nodes. It required an incision bigger than you want to imagine: over 150 staples were put into her face and neck. On my fifty-fifth birthday I went with her for her radiation treatment and cried as they bolted her to the table in a headgear that you should only see in *Star Wars*. They radiated her from four different angles, and the treatment zapped her of her energy and tested her spirit. Her cancer was particularly cruel and there were days when personally I didn't know how she carried on. I am thankful that she allowed me to be part of her life during that time. Thinking positively, she made vacation plans with her husband so they could celebrate when this was behind them. And they did exactly that.

We sometimes forget to share positive cancer stories — Barb does *not* have cancer. She beat it! Barb was diagnosed with acute lymphoblastic leukemia on what would have been my mom's birthday a few years ago (December 22). She is the same friend who was my secretary in the early '80s, went with me to all the president's hockey tournaments, and kept in touch with me when I was diagnosed. We could not have known as we laughed while we shared a glass of wine years ago that we would both enter the cancer arena at some point. I visited with her in the hospital on Christmas Day and helped her prepare for her family's visit. We decorated her IV pole and cursed cancer through our tears. Barb's mom, Addie, is such a wonderful lady and I love her. Barb and I once took our mothers to their appointments at Sunnybrook on the same day (her mother had been diagnosed as well) and arranged to take them to McDonald's for lunch afterwards. Addie told me during Barb's illness how hard it was for her to watch her "Barbie" battle cancer and how very proud she was of her baby. Barb is much younger than her siblings. As I listened to

Addie I could only imagine that my mother felt exactly the same way watching her daughter battle cancer. It made me even closer to both Barb and her mom. It is so important to celebrate victories in the cancer arena.

Often when someone talks about retiring they worry about losing contact with those who have been important to them over the years. I have found that it is possible to maintain those contacts and I have also found they become even more meaningful when these people are not part of your day-to-day life. I still get together with my colleagues from Bell — managers, executives, and more than anyone else, the guys from my Installation and Repair team.

I am always serious about my New Year's resolutions, and I try to execute the major ones by the end of March. It's the business side of me coming out — make the resolution and then make it happen, and do it early in the year. At the end of 2000 one of my major resolutions for the New Year was to rid myself of my father's nose. I first considered this when I was forty, but couldn't find a surgeon with whom I felt confident. At forty-five I was battling cancer, and by fifty I was happy to be alive. As I approached my fifty-fifth birthday the operation seemed the perfect gift — my version of "Freedom 55." I would banish a ghost from my past.

It took me over a year to find the surgeon who was right for me, and that was Dr. William Middleton. A friend went with me for the initial consultation and then I went on my own until I had made all of my decisions. I would have my face "refreshed" at the same time that I had my "nose job." Writing about cosmetic surgery is somewhat difficult to do. After enduring cancer surgery, this operation would be purely for vanity, and who wants to openly admit they are vain? I wanted to have the surgery and didn't want to invent stories that were untrue if someone should ask me questions. After all my questions were answered and I spent some quiet time reflecting on my decision, the date was set. My family understood and was supportive. I told a few close friends in advance and they were both curious about the procedure and supportive of my decision.

The surgery went well and I chose to remain at the clinic overnight under the watchful eye of nurse Mary. Dr. Middleton had told me that one other person would be staying at the clinic that night as well. I awakened during the night, heard a man's voice and said, "Hey Mary, things are looking up. Do I hear a man in my room?" The voice from the next bed said, "Hi Carol Ann, that's the good news — the bad news is I am eighty-one years old." I saw him in the morning and we should all look so good at eighty-one! Later during that night I awakened again and instantly thought "Oh my God, I'm blind." I couldn't see a thing. My mind raced to a few years earlier when I had laser surgery to correct my vision. Maybe I forgot to tell the doctor about that; maybe you can't combine these two types of surgery. I called nurse Mary immediately. She removed the ice pack from my eyes and said, "Yes dear, what is it?" I could now see clearly; I hadn't realized there had been an ice pack on my face.

I left the next day and checked in with some friends of mine. If I can offer any advice to someone considering cosmetic surgery it would be to bunk in for a few days with someone who has been through it. They know exactly what to expect, and can help you with all the anxieties as you go through the recovery stages. Seven days after surgery I returned to the clinic to have the cast removed from my nose. I tried to think of my friend Pat who had to have all those staples in her face and neck following her cancer surgery. If she could get through that, surely I could handle having a little cast taken off my nose, and a few stitches attended to. No such luck. I fainted as soon as the cast was removed! The good news was that there was hardly any bruising left, and while there was still considerable swelling in my nose I liked the look of the new me. As I gingerly stepped down the back steps of the clinic, I heard a voice say, "Excuse me, are you Carol Ann Cole?" I didn't want to turn around and all I could think was "God, this can't be happening to me." But I looked at the woman and said, yes I was Carol Ann. The woman told me she was a breast cancer survivor, owned one of the Comfort Hearts, and was glad to finally meet me! I thanked her but explained it was obviously not a good time to chat. As I got in the car, I said to my friend, "Can you believe it? I can't get away from Comfort Heart stories even when I am hiding out!" We both laughed all the way home and I marvelled at the situations the Comfort Heart Initiative has gotten me into.

Given that I was now recovering very well from the surgery, I turned my full attention to my back injury. Just before my surgery, I had been moving furniture and felt a sharp pain in my back. When I tried to walk my one foot started to drag, and I couldn't figure out what I'd done. Being totally unfamiliar with back or hip injuries I sought considerable medical advice. CT scans and an MRI confirmed there was no back injury, but I had developed a condition called "foot drop" that would take time to correct. I guess if I had realized the extent of my injury I may have kept my nose out of it for a while.

I might have gotten rid of his nose, but Dad is still in my life and I visit him in the nursing home as often as I can. I forgave him years ago, not so much for him, but so that I could move forward with my own life. We never talk about the past — he is blind and confined to a wheelchair — but in many ways he has not changed at all.

Moving home to Nova Scotia has brought me so much peace. I love living near the ocean and I love the people here. I've always been a Maritimer at heart. Shortly after moving home, I was the guest speaker at the Middleton Regional High School 49th graduation exercises. As we filed out of the over-crowded and overheated auditorium, one very elderly lady approached me and said, "Dear, we are very proud of you here in Middleton. You can go anywhere you like, but you belong to us."

Home is where the heart is.

I have been very fortunate and have experienced so much — I know without question that I can learn as much travel-ling on a bus as I can in a limo. Additionally I can learn as much in a garage as I can in a corporate boardroom. When the hem came out of that camel-coloured ostrich suit en route to a president's meeting in Montreal I learned that gum could be used instead of needle and thread in a pinch and worked as well on a $2,500 suit as it did on my jeans.

I still love hearing stories from people who've bought Comfort Hearts. Of all the Comfort Heart stories I could share, perhaps the most meaningful was from Maureen Hayden. The Canadian Auto Workers had invited me to speak at the International Women's Day Annual Information Fair in Windsor. Maureen spoke before me and reduced everyone to tears with her personal story of hope and dreams. She was wearing her Comfort Heart with "Maureen" inscribed on the back — not because it was her name, but because it was also the name of the technician who discovered the lump in her breast at the local breast screening clinic. Maureen is of Scottish descent and shared with the audience a wonderful tradition in her family. Each woman, at birth, is given a treasure trove — a box to hold her treasures throughout her life. Annually, or whenever the family gathers, the women all bring their treasure troves. The oldest woman is treated like a rock star — she has the most stories to tell and the most treasures in her box. Everyone gathers at her feet listening to her stories relating to her many treasures. Maureen's dream is to be one hundred years old, with everyone sitting at her feet and listening as she takes her Comfort Heart out of her treasure box. She will tell the story of how she came to have a Comfort Heart, and one of the young family members at her feet will say, "Is it true that women used to die from breast cancer?" Maureen will be able to confidently reply, "That's true, honey, they used to. But no more, because we have found a cure for breast cancer."

That's my dream, too.

Epilogue

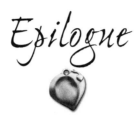

*F*ew circumstances in my life have prepared me for the contents of the envelope I received on December 11, 2000. I had just completed a Canadian Breast Cancer Research Initiative meeting, and chose to walk back to my loft, enjoying the beauty of an early evening snowfall. When I reached the lobby, I chatted with the girls at the front desk as they handed me an envelope that had just arrived. I absent-mindedly glanced at the label, which was marked "Confidential" in bold letters, with the address Government House, 1 Sussex Drive, Ottawa. My curiosity was piqued as I opened the envelope, and when I caught a glimpse of the Rideau Hall letterhead I immediately hurried to my apartment. I opened the door, put my briefcase down, turned on the light, and with my coat still on, unfolded the letter and read:

**Dear Mrs. Cole, [my first thought was, they got *that* wrong!]
We are pleased to inform you that the Advisory Council of
the Order of Canada has recommended to the Governor
General that you be appointed a Member of the Order of
Canada.**

The letter went on to say that the information was strictly
confidential and I must respect that. Of course, I immediately
called my son and then my sisters. It was a very hard secret
to keep, so it was a great relief when they announced it for-
mally. On Friday, February 16, along with fifty-five other
Canadians, I was named to the Order of Canada of Voluntary
Service. The full list of names was published in the *Globe and
Mail*, and the response to my nomination was overwhelming.

My phone rang off the hook for the day and I could barely
keep up with the e-mails that I received. The congratulatory
notes poured in from former colleagues at Bell, good friends,
and all the people who helped make the Comfort Heart
Initiative happen.

In many ways it was very appropriate that James was the
family member accompanying me to the Order of Canada ceremony. You can only bring one person with you, but for me
the decision was an easy one — I knew James was the one.
He was very excited when he found out I had been nominated
and his anticipation grew in the months leading up to the
actual event. For him, it was the culmination of all the things
he has watched me do and be recognized for over the years.

James and I flew to Ottawa the day before the ceremony
and spent the evening having a long talk over dinner at Hy's
Steakhouse — a place I had been many times in my career

at Bell, but never with my son. We reminisced about the time we had spent in Ottawa — the first condo we purchased and how different this dinner was from earlier years when James would order the Number Four from the Ponderosa menu. We also talked about how hard it was to only bring one person to this momentous ceremony — although James had his own view on the matter: "Actually, I think this is the way it should be," he said. "It was only the two of us for many years and I like it that way for this event — just you and me." It was a great ending to the dinner and we both went back to the hotel in a jubilant mood.

The morning of Thursday, May 31, started with a promising message — my horoscope for the day began with this sentence: "Affairs of the heart will go extremely well today . . ." I spent the early part of the afternoon getting ready. I had chosen to wear a black Jil Sander dress I had purchased twelve years before for a Bell corporate function. It was simple, yet slightly funky with a jagged hemline; most importantly, it signified my style. At the last moment I realized I would not be able to wear the strappy gold sandals I had purchased for the occasion because of my foot drop. I wore my clunky black sandals instead and just hoped that no one would film my feet.

The one thing that really struck me about the whole Order of Canada ceremony is the formality and protocol — it makes everything seem more momentous. Shortly after arriving at Rideau Hall, James and I were separated into the different groups of guests and honorees. We were given explicit instructions on how to behave in front of the Governor General, and how to receive the award. It was very exciting, but I began to get nervous as we lined up in alphabetical order to enter the hall. With the sounds of the Woodwind Quintet of the Canadian Forces Central Band in the background, we proceeded down the aisle and took our seat. Her Excellency The Right Honourable Adrienne Clarkson and His Excellency John Ralston Saul entered as the Vice Regal salute was played, and I felt she was looking directly at me as she walked in (of course I'm sure everyone else thought the same thing).

I was tenth in line to be called to the front, and with all due respect to the nine people receiving the Order of Canada before me, I was not paying attention at all. My heart was beating wildly as I heard them announce my name. As I stepped forward, I thought about the 160,000 Canadians who held the Comfort Heart and all it represented. And as the announcer recited my bio, my thoughts turned to my mother — the inspiration behind the Comfort Heart Initiative. The entire time I stood before the Governor General felt very surreal; it was almost like I was moving in slow motion as she shook my hand and I heard all of the cameras clicking, and flashes bouncing off the walls. It was over very quickly and I sat through the rest of the ceremony trying to focus my attention on the remaining recipients. At the end, when everyone stood to sing the National Anthem I had a private chuckle as I thought about my imaginary childhood hero, Gloria Sandfree.

Immediately after the ceremony, CTV News interviewed me and once again my thoughts turned to Mom. She would have loved all of the attention I was receiving, and I wished she could have been there to stand with James while the media interviews were happening. I imagined her and James would have found humour in all the hoopla, and I could hear her commenting about my "foot-drop" shoes.

We were then ushered into a beautiful room for a sump-tuous dinner. The meal was wonderful, but the most memorable part for me was the conversation. I was unprepared for, and totally humbled by the number of people who approached me to talk about their own Comfort Heart stories — both Order of Canada recipients and guests. Once again I was struck by the power these pewter hearts have over so many people.

James had to leave right after the dinner to make it to work the next morning and he told me how proud he was of me as I kissed him goodbye. After he left a few people approached me to tell me how much they had enjoyed talking with James over the course of the evening. One woman pointed out that my greatest accomplishment had to be raising a son like James, and I couldn't agree with her more.

The Governor General had announced that the halls and rooms of Rideau Hall would be open for us to tour after dinner. I thought of how my mother would have loved to have been there for a private tour of Rideau Hall. She adored visiting the Parliament buildings in Ottawa. As I walked through the splen-dorous rooms, I thought about the road that had brought me to this point in my life. I know that if I had not lost my mother to cancer, I would not likely be standing in Rideau Hall at that moment — and it is a very bittersweet feeling to honour your mother after she has passed away. At the same time, if Mom had not insisted I move away from home, had faltered at her decision thirty-seven years ago, then I also would not have achieved the things I have in my life. I still continue to learn from her.

Now I have a tiny snowflake pin that will continue to inspire me in all of the decisions I make in my life. Each time

I look at my Order of Canada medal I am reminded that one person truly can make a difference. Dreams do come true if you have the power to believe and stay positive. I will always have the profound hope that this award, and this book, will inspire others to give back — from the heart.

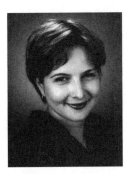

Anjali Kapoor is an online journalist for MochaSofa.ca, a women's web portal, based in Toronto. She has covered a variety of women's issues over the years as a lifestyle writer for CANOE.ca and as a freelancer to publications such as *Homemaker's* magazine, *Chatelaine,* and the *National Post.*

Ordering Comfort Hearts

Thanks a million!

Yes, it's true. We have raised over one million dollars for cancer research through the sale of Comfort Hearts.

Around the world there are over 160,000 people who have joined my team that I affectionately call the "Holders of the Heart." They joined by making a purchase of a Comfort Heart — and you can too.

To order, you can call OceanArt Pewter at 1-800-407-4436, or visit their Web site at **www.oceanartpewter.com**
To order directly through mail please send your cheque or money order ($10 per heart) payable to the Comfort Heart Initiative to:

Comfort Heart Initiative
Box 27013
Halifax, Nova Scotia
B3H 4M8

Additionally, you can reach me directly through my Web site at **www.carolanncole.com**